RECONSTRUCTING NURSING:
BEYOND ART AND SCIENCE

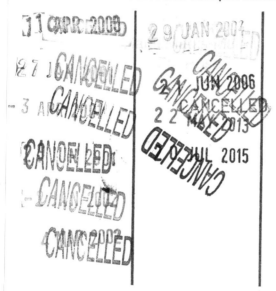
PUBLISHED IN ASSOCIATION WITH THE RCN

London Philadelphia Toronto Sydney Tokyo

BAILLIÈRE TINDALL
An imprint of Harcourt Publishers Limited

© 1997 Baillière Tindall

First published 1997
  Reprinted 1999

ISBN 07020 2000 1

British Library Cataloguing in Publication Data
A catalogue record for this book is available from the British Library

Library of Congress Cataloging in Publication Data
A catalog record for this book is available from the Library of Congress

Printed in China
NPCC/02

Contents

Contributors

Diane Marks-Maran BSc, RGN, Dip N (Lond), RNT
Wolfson School of Health and Science, Thames Valley University, 32–38 Uxbridge Road, Ealing, London W5 2BS

♦

David Parker MA, BN, RMN, RGN, Cert Ed, FETC
School of Health, University of Greenwich, Elizabeth Raybould Centre, Bow Arrow Lane, Dartford, Kent, DA2 6PJ

♦

Pat Rose RGN, RSCN, MSc, BSc, Dip N (Lond), Cert Ed
School of Health, University of Greenwich, Avery Hill Campus, Bexley Road, London SE9 2PQ

♦

Verena Tschudin BSc (Hons), RN, RM, Dip Counselling
University of East London, Romford Road, London E15 4LZ

♦

Professor Jean Watson RN, PLD, FAAN
Center for Human Caring, School of Nursing, University of Colorado, 4200 East Ninth Avenue, Box C288, Denver, Colorado 80262, USA

Acknowledgements

It is difficult to decide who to acknowledge and thank for making it possible for us to create this book. We could write a full chapter about all those who have helped us along the way, but that would hardly be practical. Instead we want to say a particular thank you to the following:

To Sarah James, the nursing publisher at Baillière Tindall, for her excitement from the day we came to see her with the seed of an idea, throughout its germination and gestation, to the birth of the book.

To Sally Thomson, who facilitated our reflective thinking, as we undertook a Reflective Practice module at the Royal College of Nursing in 1993. In fact it was there that we, the editors, met each other, and where we inadvertently sowed the first seed of the book. Thanks Sally for being there from the beginning, and for letting us know we could do it.

To Jean Watson, David Parker, and Verena Tschudin, who each contributed chapters to the book. It was you three who helped turn the idea into reality.

To Nicky Cadisch, Sharmila Patel, Dee Cunnington and Richard Horner, who did the practical things; typing, re-typing, keeping computers and printers going. Your patience is exemplary. Likewise, to our colleagues, who supported us through the ups and downs of the process, and our moods associated with these.

Thanks also to all those countless people, many of whose names appear on the reference list, whom we have never met, but whose ideas are, as it were, the soil nurturing the seed.

Finally to you, our readers. It's up to you to scatter the seed amongst those we care for, our patients.

Di Marks-Maran
Pat Rose
1996

The Beginning . . . .

In *Reconstructing Nursing: Beyond Art and Science* we are attempting to go beyond some traditional ways of understanding nursing. You will therefore find this book quite different from many others which explore a variety of current and future nursing issues.

Firstly, the use of language has been carefully considered, moving from third person (objective = science) to first person (subjective = art). This is deliberate, as a way of using language as a metaphor for the message we are trying to deliver. In addition, out of respect for nursing tradition, and accepting the risk that we might be labelled as 'politically incorrect', we have chosen to call those whom we nurse, *patients*.

Secondly, there is a recurring theme which weaves its way like a tapestry throughout each chapter. This theme is the theme of the cube. In this book the cube has come to be another metaphor. Each face of the cube represents a different paradigm or world view of nursing. As you hold a cube in your hands and turn it around, there are always faces of that cube which are clearly visible, faces which can be partially visible and always at least one face which is hidden. No matter what you do (unless you use mirrors!) you can never see all the faces of the cube at the same time. The top and bottom faces of the cube represent opposites in nursing: art and science; theory and practice; professional and vocational; thinking and doing; knowledge and action. Each chapter refers to the cube in its unique way and the final chapter suggests a new face for the cube – a new world view of nursing.

The third aspect of this book which may appear to be a little different is the inclusion of a conversation between each chapter. In these conversations, the next chapter has a discussion with the previous chapter, highlighting and summarizing the previous, linking the two and introducing the next chapter. The conversations were born out of the discussions, telephone calls, correspondence and e-mails we had with each other and with David, Verena and Jean who wrote three of the chapters.

For too long science and art have been seen in a dualist way as opposites in conflict. This book tries to demonstrate that opposites are not in conflict but are connected by an energy flowing between them. The conversations between chapters tap into that connective energy.

This is a book of ideas and possibilities, suggestions and discussion. It is not an answer but a journey. To quote Richard Bach (1978):

everything in this book may be wrong

Chapter 1

NURSING ART AND SCIENCE: LITERATURE AND DEBATE

David Parker

The nature of nursing and its knowledge base seem to be somewhat elusive phenomena which have stretched the minds of nurse practitioners, scholars and researchers over many decades. This chapter includes a selective, and somewhat personal, review of the literature in an attempt to raise some of the critical issues for debate and to identify the factors which may well determine the nature of the profession of nursing in the 21st century.

A brief introduction to the literature on the nature of knowledge and its possible effects on nursing's quest for identity and self-acceptance as a practice discipline is followed by two main sections. The first section is designed to assist the reader to explore the concept of nursing as an art. It becomes apparent that there is a requirement for conceptual clarity in terms of nursing art: a need that may not have received the appropriate recognition or attention until fairly recently, despite the fact that nursing scholars have written about the concept over many decades. It is still evident that status differences between art and science remain, to the possible detriment of patient-centred humanistic nursing practice. The second section, an exploration of nursing as a science, includes a discussion on the requirement for research which advances knowledge and theory development, together with a critical review of the various scientific paradigms. Ways in which various scholars have attempted to define and classify nursing science are presented in an attempt to identify some of the areas which may require further discussion and debate within the profession, in order to advance knowledge that will be useful to patients/clients, practising nurses, nurse educators and students.

The reader may detect a change of style between the two main sections. This is a deliberate ploy to demonstrate more effectively differences in the language, as well as the nature, of art and science in nursing. The second section is followed by a discussion of the nature of reflection and its potential for the development of professional artistry, as well as a foundation for empirical, practice-based science.

◆

APPROACHES TO KNOWLEDGE, THEORY AND PRACTICE

It is often said that nursing is more an art than a science, with art being linked, through ignorance and prejudice, to untested practise and strongly held beliefs which are fundamentally inferior to scientific, validated knowledge or 'facts'. Possibly the most critical debate in the literature is on the nature of facts and theories. There appears to be no unified view: distinctions between fact and theory remain hair-splitting, unclear and confusing (Meleis, 1991). Polit and Hungler (1991) describe facts as being empirical, in other words information that can be experienced through the human senses. Facts are verified through researchers' observations of the world and, as such, do not require theory. Such research has its limitations, however, since individual perceptions are important, particularly in the human sciences such as nursing. From the perspective of the new paradigm researchers in social science (Reason and Rowen, 1981) and feminist researchers such as Oakley (1982) and Burman (1990), there is no such thing as objective, value free science. All researchers should therefore make clear their theoretical perspectives, or faces on the cube, so that readers are able to grasp the assumptions underpinning the research and thereby be aware of its uses and possible limitations.

Webb (1992a), in a debate entitled 'what is nursing?', describes the recent efforts to re-define nursing. She suggests that many nursing writers have encouraged a move away from the traditional medically dominated approach, towards psychosocial care and forming relationships with patients. She highlights particular conceptual frameworks of nursing, such as those of Roy (1981) and Orem (1985), and believes they have succeeded in keeping a more even balance than Roper, Logan and Tierney (1985).

As a nurse lecturer, I have read many students' essays berating Roper, Logan and Tierney for their medically oriented, materialist, mechanistic, reductionist approach. I feel we too easily discard something which is easy to comprehend, straightforward and actually works in conjunction with medical practice, in favour of an approach such as that of Roy, which may be much more difficult to implement. Roper, Logan and Tierney actually do include psychosocial aspects within their framework, but the tendency is to ignore those factors which influence the patient's activities of living whilst carrying out assessment and care planning. It is certainly the case that this oft vilified 'model' is utilized, admittedly with varying degrees of enthusiasm and success, in numerous clinical settings and specialisms throughout the United Kingdom.

Webb (1992a) criticizes Salvage's (1990) concept of 'new nursing': the use of models as bases for individualized care plans which focus on patients' psychological and social problems or needs as well as the physical problems linked to their medical diagnoses and treatment. Salvage rightly points out that the patient's immediate concern tends to be the relief of pain and discomfort, not the development of meaningful relationships with their primary nurses. Webb acknowledges the work of Campbell (1984) and Oakley (1984), both of whom are sceptical about the closeness of the nurse–patient relationship. She concludes the debate with a plea for us not to lose the traditional emphasis on physical care and comfort in the struggle to humanize care and make it more responsive to patients' supposed wishes for greater involvement in decisions about their own health and treatment (Webb, 1992a).

The conclusion which may be drawn from this introduction to the art and science debate is that nurses need to be aware of the strengths and limitations of traditional and new approaches to knowledge, theory and practice so that nursing may become an activity which is delivered in a humanistic way, critically integrating within practice the richness of the wide range of perspectives available.

Chinn (1994) describes the opening of doors of possibility by Carper (1978), who identified four patterns of knowing in nursing. These patterns of knowing: empirical; ethical; personal; and aesthetic, have frequently been utilized in scholarly work over the preceding 17 years: examples can be seen in numerous recent articles on the nature of nursing (Rose and Parker, 1994; Sweeney, 1994; Behi and Nolan, 1995). Chinn suggests that the value of Carper's work lies in the resultant widespread recognition that nurses and nursing depend on, and need, forms of knowledge in addition to that provided by empirical science. Chinn suggests that philosophical enquiry has become recognized and valued in nursing, but that methods involving the non-discursive realm of knowing, such as art and aesthetics, have been slower to evolve and develop. She suggests that these approaches to the understanding of nursing are different from the methods used in the more familiar world of empirics and that they have unique criteria by which their worth or adequacy is judged. She highlights the possibilities for challenging the status quo and for bringing to awareness the possibilities that are not yet widely recognized: '. . . esthetic inquiry is beginning to raise interesting questions about what it means to know, about the fundamental nature of "science" as we have known it and as it could become in the future' (Chinn, 1994, p.viii).

A word of caution is offered by Shaw (1993), who questions Fawcett's (1984a) belief that empiricism may be incompatible with nursing's humanistic and holistic aims. She believes that the rejection of quantitative research methods due to fear of dehumanizing patients with reductionist methods would be an epistemological error. Like the students, in their nursing models essays, who berate Roper, Logan and Tierney, nurses are at risk of rejecting the empirical method which has undoubtedly advanced medical science and informed the practice of nursing.

◆

NURSING AS AN ART

Shaw (1993) calls for an era of theory development and refinement, 'from a rich tapestry of theoretical perspectives and research methodologies' to fulfil nursing's quest for identity as well as for self-acceptance as a practice discipline. It is this practice element which in the past has been viewed as nursing art.

It has been suggested that art is a skill or craft which is not instinctual, but is learned, also that it carries connotations of creativity and beauty (Rose and Parker, 1994). Harrison-Barbet (1990) thus poses the question as to whether there may be criteria that must be fulfilled for something to be considered art, or that it may simply be a matter of subjective opinion. Rose and Parker (1994) give the examples in nursing of practice of a novice and an experienced nurse, or between a caring and a uncaring nurse. They give further examples of bad art, defined by Harrison-Barbet (1990) as that which has the effect of corrupting consciousness, as flippant nurses provoking anxiety in a patient whilst seeking to promote humour, or using an interpersonal relationship to gratify their own needs, rather than those of the patient. They conclude their paper by arguing for the acceptance of tacit knowledge and intuition within nursing. They further suggest that 'nursing as an integration of art and science may be used to develop nursing creatively for the benefit of patients . . . who receive nursing care and medical treatment through their perceived world' (Rose and Parker, 1994). I believe that this argument is one to which many nurses from all specialisms will be able to relate. We all know an uncaring nurse when we see one – we do not need a battery of empirical tests and carefully designed research projects to 'prove' it. As an experienced nurse I know when I am doing a good job, when an interaction is going well or when a student is honing and developing new skills under my supervision. Much of this knowledge is personal – it does not emanate from books, journals, lectures or academic conferences. Rose and Parker (1994) appeal for the intuitive, the creative; yes, even the *artistic* in nursing.

According to Johnson (1994), however, there is need for conceptual clarity regarding nursing art. She presents the findings of a dialectical study based on the works of 41 nursing scholars published between 1860 and 1992. Her analysis revealed five distinct conceptualizations, which can be identified as the art of:

Grasping meaning in patient encounters

As a mental health nurse I derive meaning from my ability to empathize with a patient and to facilitate the development of mutual understanding within each unique situation. This ability is derived from personal knowledge and expertise acquired over many years of

7

nursing practice. It is an art that requires not only knowledge and expertise, but intuition and the desire to care for and help another human being. This motivation to care is not only essential for grasping meaning but also a requirement when I expand my art to include Johnson's second conceptualization.

Establishing a meaningful connection with the patient

This can be exemplified by examining the process described by Peplau (1952) of the interpersonal relationship in nursing. By utilizing the four phases of orientation, identification, exploitation and resolution I am able to collaborate with the patient in the agreement of mutually understood goals through which we may both grow and learn. This meaningful connection is only possible by virtue of my desire and ability to relate to the patient's situation and the art of connecting between one individual and another. As the relationship develops, goals converge into the working phase of exploitation, to appropriately diverge within the resolution phase as the connection is therapeutically diminished.

Skilfully performing nursing activities

An example scenario from general nursing will exemplify the art of skilful nursing intervention. A patient is lying in bed after a surgical procedure: is in pain, anxious and looks and feels unwashed, unkempt and somewhat unloved. The art of nursing is clearly demonstrated in the almost miraculous transformation into a clean, comfortable, less anxious and well informed human being who is beginning to assume control over their life once more after feeling lost in a world of technology, pain, confusion and helplessness. I am sure that all caring, expert nurses can relate to this scenario and think of countless times when they have marvelled at the transformations possible through skilful application of nursing art. The situation is always different, the patient problems diverse, but the end result of patient and nurse satisfaction and the achievement of mutually agreed nursing outcomes is what really makes the job worthwhile.

Rationally determining an appropriate course of nursing action

Nursing science cannot, in itself, enable me to determine rationally the most appropriate interventions for a particular patient in a unique and ever changing situation. Knowledge derived from research needs to be transformed into personal knowledge through its application to countless situations in nursing practice. By testing out different approaches in many different situations I am able to transform rather arid textbook knowledge into fruitful expertise. There is a considerable literature on the theory and practice of reflection arising from scholars such as Argyris and Schon (1974) and Boud, Keogh and Walker (1985). Practitioners such as Johns (1992) have demonstrated how the theoretical concepts introduced by scholars may be understood and subsequently utilized in practice. As a nursing lecturer I frequently use the variety of models of reflection currently available so that I can help students to understand the reality of practical reflection. This may assist them to not only improve their practice, but also to write reflectively in course assignments and reflective journals.

Morally conducting one's nursing practice

It is my view that no research or textbook knowledge can adequately prepare me for the plethora of moral dilemmas I encounter in everyday nursing practice. The way I see the world and my subsequent actions are influenced by my own and my profession's codes of conduct. My stage of moral development is such that I have progressed from the position of needing guidelines imposed largely by others. Expert nurses operate within a moral code which reflects their individuality and their willingness to accept personal and professional accountability for their practice.

I am able to accept Johnson's conceptualizations for two main reasons. On the intellectual level, I am able to understand and exemplify them. On the personal level they intuitively appear right and of critical importance to my practice as a nurse. Johnson (1994) suggests that science alone will not solve all of the problems of nursing: it is essential to consider the manner in which knowledge, judgement and skill are used in the clinical setting. 'These phenomena fall generally under the rubric of art of nursing. Ultimately, an understanding of nursing art will further an understanding of how excellence can best be pursued and achieved in nursing practice'. Johnson hopes that by identifying distinct conceptions of nursing art, productive debate and analysis among nursing scholars will be facilitated.

According to Hampton (1994) a wealth of untapped knowledge exists, embedded in the expert practice of clinicians. She suggests that expertise more closely relates to the artistic than the empirical. She cites the work of Thompson, Ryan and Kitzman (1990) on the characteristics of expertise, listing these as quality decision making, intuition, knowledge, adept psychomotor skills and clinical specialization. It may appear obvious that experts require empirics, ethics, aesthetics and personal knowledge to achieve these characteristics. Hampton, however, suggests that experts do not need to rely on conscious reasoning in practice as often as novices do, thus being less aware of reasons for their actions. This automatic response, or feeling, may be labelled intuition. 'Intuitive perception, or the immediate knowing of something without using conscious reason, leads to a different sense of understanding than what is possible through reason alone' (Hampton, 1994). She further describes intuition as a sophisticated form of reasoning that is acquired by the expert over years of learning and thus falls largely within the domain of art in nursing. Citing the important work of Benner (1984) in articulating the knowledge embedded in the practice of expert nurses, she advocates that nurses need to have a continued focus on how the concept of expertise relates to the essence of nursing. This, she suggests, will help nurses to continue to value their artistic abilities.

Gendron (1994) uses the fascinating analogy of tapestry to explore artistic nursing activities, describing the warp as acontextual knowledge and skills, available resources and agency policies; the weft as the creative pattern of care. She further describes the warp as a background structure involving scientific facts, conceptual ideas, technical skills and the assessing, planning, implementing and evaluating skill components of the nursing process. This background structure also incorporates nursing's professional mandate and role. The weft of care is defined as 'a creative pattern . . . woven on the warp strings of constraints, knowledge and skills' (Gendron, 1994). She suggests that art in nursing evolves: it is not a calculated construction. She asserts that the aesthetic pattern is paramount in nursing, suggesting that the weft has the qualities of balance, harmony, rhythm, tone and unity. Gendron suggests that one needs to match nursing actions to another person by attuning to, and synchronizing with, the person being cared for, requiring an intuitive grasp or whole understanding. 'The analogy of warp and weft can help nurses think about how a structured framework for practice is combined with creative, individualized care for each person – the essence of nursing art' (Gendron, 1994). I concur with this thesis. Who can teach me to match my nursing actions with another person as described above? I learn to do this through observing 'good' nurses, through testing different approaches in real patient-focused situations, through intuition; but primarily as a result of the desire to help someone, to care for them and to enable them to cope with their illness or disability, or to recover fully and perhaps enjoy an increased level of wellness and quality of life. Motivation to care is something which cannot be taught, nor can it be gained from empirical research projects. It can, however, be nurtured.

Darbyshire (1994) suggests that of all of nursing's clichés, nursing as an art and science is the least reflected in reality. He describes the characterization of nursing by the desire to establish professional and academic credibility through an alignment with science. He traces the moves of nursing's academics from hospitals to academic settings which, he suggests, were accompanied by a strong reliance upon empiricism and behaviourism. He decries the domination of the rational-calculative thinking of the scientific method in nursing education. 'Under such a template of thought, the art of nursing and other more meditative, contemplative, and aesthetic modes of thinking and engaging with the world have been at best marginalised and at worst excluded' (Darbyshire, 1994). He suggests that nurses can best gain insight and understanding into dimensions of the human condition and the lived experiences of illness, suffering, dying, healing, pain and disability through study and dialogue related to poetry, art, music, film and other media.

He further describes the use of Frida Kahlo's paintings in a course for students to experience new ways of thinking, learning and understanding in relation to the lived experience of human suffering. Darbyshire (1994) adds that the art of nursing cannot be promoted merely by stating that nursing is an art. 'For nursing, to realise its potential as a creative, healing art, as opposed to a mere customer satisfaction technique, nurses need to create alternative ways of thinking and of understanding human experience that are not exclusively instrumental and technologic'. He presents a powerful argument for a balanced curriculum to enable nurses to fulfil their full potential. He cites Bevis (1989) who asserts that science may give us the tools for curing, but it is the humanities which give us the tools for caring.

Merkle Sorrell (1994) furthers the debate about aesthetics in nursing. She suggests that creative imagination is needed for discovery in science. She identifies characteristics of aesthetic knowledge as creativity, discovery, fluidity, openness, appreciation, expressivity and imagination as critical in nursing science. She advocates the process of writing for nurses to recapture important subjective experiences in nursing and suggests that, as we reflect intuitively on these experiences, we create insights and interpretations that promote aesthetic ways of knowing. Merkle Sorrell suggests the following strategies, to foster aesthetic thoughtfulness in nursing:

1. Incorporating expressive and poetic writing into nursing curricula.
2. Writing reflectively in a nursing journal to serve as a bridge to new enquiries and understanding of nursing traditions.
3. Interdisciplinary writing to identify common understanding between health professionals.
4. Integrating aesthetic patterns of knowing with empirical, ethical and personal patterns of knowing in nursing research.
5. Exploring stylistic aspects of language, such as metaphor and poetry, to evoke thought and enhance meaning in textual representation of qualitative research.

Merkle Sorrell (1994) puts forward a very strong case for the use of the writing process as a valuable medium for aesthetic knowing. She makes a plea that the desire to build a strong scientific base for nursing should not be allowed to obscure the more elusive aesthetic underpinnings. The debate on nursing art, although emotive in parts, remains compelling. I would like to reiterate that the teaching and learning of nursing students does not have to be haphazard and largely dependent on their levels of caring, creativity and motivation. I have demonstrated that nursing may be studied in a rigorous manner, using a wide variety of valid, reliable methods. This 'nursing' may be defined as the skilful art of integrating personal, aesthetic, ethical and empirical knowledge into the unique and ever changing situation within which the nurse, patient and significant others find themselves. The elusive factor seems to be the acknowledgement, by nurses themselves, of the critical importance of the art of the discipline, rather than its academic advancement and acceptance by the scientific community.

Brink (1993) uses the analogy of the artist to facilitate understanding of the relationship between art and science in nursing. She suggests that, like the artist, the nurse has some inherent talent for nursing which needs to be developed and perfected through practice. As all artists need to know something about their art, so do nurses need to know about their nursing. Brink (1993) defines the science of nursing as its knowledge base: 'Just as a dancer or a painter needs to know the science behind the dance or painting, so too the nurse needs to know the science behind the artistry of nursing'. She reflects on the critical importance of science to a knowledge and appreciation of what has gone on before, how nurses have solved problems and what explanations they have offered to underpin the recommended behaviour or interventions.

◆

NURSING AS A SCIENCE

The principles of scientific enquiry include research for the advancement of knowledge and theory development in an effort to provide descriptions, explanations and predictions related to phenomena (Powers and Knapp, 1990). According to Peplau (1988), the values of the scientific method are scepticism, doubt, objectivity and detachment. Reed and Procter (1993) suggest that it is these values which encourage people to view scientific knowledge as superior to other forms of knowing, and ascribe to science high academic status. Rose and Parker (1994) state that scientific enquiry is viewed as the process by which theory for nursing is primarily generated. If this is so, then the nature of scientific enquiry warrants closer examination.

Shaw (1993) traces the discipline of nursing from its historical roots through to its current perspectives and proposed future direction. She suggests that the evolving pattern of intellectual growth holds promise for the discipline of nursing through knowledge advancement based primarily upon scientific enquiry into the practice of nursing. She suggests that nurses, in a wide variety of roles and settings, continue to contribute to the discipline by clarifying the work and role of nurses in health care and advancing nursing knowledge from 'a state of haphazard, unverified thoughts to a discipline of systematically organised concepts' (Shaw, 1993). She does however state, somewhat naively, that in the 1980s nursing was accepted as a science. If the discipline of nursing is judged by its unique scientific knowledge, then it is doubtful whether it would gain acceptance as unique within much of the scientific community. In addition it may not be viewed as desirable for nursing to be conferred full acceptance as a science. This may well negate critically important areas of knowledge identified by both Carper (1978) and Chinn and Jacobs (1987), who classify nursing knowledge as empirics, ethics, personal knowledge and aesthetics. Shaw does, however, cite many nursing scholars who describe the ambiguity of nursing's definition. She describes Hardy's (1978) belief that dissent is characteristic of nursing's preparadigmatic stage of scientific development, where disputes about theory and research can be seen as a normal developmental stage during that period.

The concept of 'paradigm shift' may be a useful one to introduce here. It is suggested that scientists who work in the area of natural sciences, including medicine, share the 'perceived view'. This may be understood in terms of the perceived validity of particular types of knowledge. It may be advocated that the only 'true' or 'valid' knowledge is that which has been subjected to rigorous empirical testing utilizing mainly quantitative approaches to research.

This has been questioned in recent years by some scholars: nurses in particular have advocated the use of qualitative approaches which may yield richer data in terms of the real, lived experiences of both patients and their carers (Rose et al, 1995). If the core of nursing is the expression of caring through an interpersonal relationship, then it may be assumed that the most appropriate research methods should be drawn from phenomenology or an associated area.

Shaw (1993) suggests that nursing may not experience periods of 'normal' science, but may continue to evolve indefinitely. A straight road to a conventional paradigm may mark nursing's acceptance into the scientific community, but the advancement of nursing cannot be measured in the same way as physical, pharmacological, medical and psychological sciences. She cites writers who advocate competing theories and propose diversity and plurality. She concludes that adoption of a specific perspective is unlikely in a discipline which encompasses human behaviour. In addition 'theoretical consensus is quite unlikely in a discipline that values the role of perceptions, uniqueness and individuality in health and illness' (Shaw, 1993). Shaw includes a debate about deductive and inductive theory through a presentation of the opposing approaches within the simultaneity and totality paradigms of theory development.

Advocates of the simultaneity paradigm, theorists such as Rogers (1970), Parse (1981) and Newman (1986), espouse the theory 'of' nursing view and promote theory development that is concerned with unitary, irreducible human beings within their environments. In this paradigm, theory is drawn from nursing rather than applied to it. Theorists in the totality paradigm, such as Roy (1984) and Neuman (1982), support the theory 'for' nursing view and promote the development of speciality-focused theory for particular clinical populations. An example would be Roy (1984) who has been developing her model from 1964 until the present day, originally deriving her concept of adaptation level from earlier work by psychophysicists (Marriner-Tomey, 1994). She further utilized concepts and theory from the social sciences and later developed the humanistic base. Roy's adaptation model thus includes assumptions from systems theory, stress-adaptation theory and from humanism (Marriner-Tomey, 1994).

Shaw (1993) further suggests that, if nursing is conceptualized as a practice discipline, these theoretical perspectives are not in opposition. 'Indeed, the upcoming era of theory development and refinement from a rich tapestry of theoretical perspectives and research methodologies may fulfil nursing's quest for identify and self-acceptance as a practice discipline'.

McKenna (1993b) looks at the necessity for the development of unique theory for a science of nursing. She suggests that nursing theorists have, at times, been more concerned with achieving higher professional status than with the advancement of clinical practice. She uses the terms 'macro theory' and 'micro theory', introduced by Chinn and Jacobs (1987) and Kim (1983). A macro theory is one which is usually applied to a general area of a specific discipline, and has broadly conceptualized goals. A theory of this type would be unique to nursing. A micro theory, however, is defined as one which deals with specific and narrowly-defined phenomena. A theory of this type would tend to be more prescriptive and would utilize knowledge from other disciplines to relate to nursing practice. It appears that this classification of theory bears more than a passing resemblance to inductive and deductive theories and to the simultaneity and totality paradigms (Parse, 1987).

'Although nursing knowledge is not unique, the application of that knowledge into practice is unique. Nursing must therefore have a unique form of theory that reflects this' (McKenna, 1993b). McKenna calls for unique nursing theories that systematize both knowledge and practice. She concludes by suggesting that, in the drive towards developing a science of nursing, we must not develop nursing theory that promotes rational, systematic practice that can be measured tested and quantified, to the detriment of other unique aspects of nursing that cannot be measured in terms of productivity and are therefore not seen as scientific. She gives the example of the concept of caring, which, in terms of nursing behaviour, is highly valued by the patient, but often undervalued or not acknowledged by the theorist.

Orem's grand theory of self-care deficit in nursing was first published in 1971. It has been widely accepted and utilized in nursing practice, but does not generally include in its usage any overt significant requirement for the nurse to be a caring person. It may be suggested that Orem's professional/ technical language assumes that the nurse is a highly educated expert in the professional activity of nursing (Orem, 1985). The requirements for a warm, caring, empathetic, non-judgmental approach, although implicitly present, tend to be lost in all the academic jargon. This represents a return to the assertion that nursing and nursing science must reflect the composite of empirical, ethical, aesthetic and personal knowledge, not all of which may fulfil scientific criteria of being empirically testable or embrace the values of scepticism, doubt, objectivity and detachment. Some nursing theorists appear to have embraced the knowledge and language of empirical science, to the potential detriment of focused, humanistic patient care.

Kim (1993) postulates that the major concerns expressed in the literature regarding nursing science arise from questions related to the type of sciences and the sort of scientific methods appropriate to nursing. She acknowledges the sector of scientific population that advocates a unified approach, but supports the position of philosophical and methodological pluralism. She acknowledges her earlier (1989) work which includes the assertion that the nature of the products of sciences is influenced by the scientist's view regarding methods, definitions of knowledge structure, aims of the discipline and focus of attention. She stresses the crucial importance of the scientist's coherent articulation of position or perspectives in terms of philosophy, theory and method. Kim rejects the usual distinctions pitting qualitative against quantitative in contrasting various approaches such as empiricism versus interpretivism. She presents a bipolar framework combining three-level dimensions of philosophy, theory generation and methodology.

Level one (philosophical orientation) includes two major positions in ontology and epistemology of interest to nursing science: scientific realism and relativism. Realism represents a position in which science helps us to understand and explain the world/reality through networks, models, metaphors and idealizations corresponding to the real world. The position of medical science in terms of its view of the person as a complex of interrelated systems, each of which can be scrutinized, may be described as realism. Relativism represents a position in which science helps us to understand and explain the world within the context of given circumstances which cannot be transcended. Relativism, espoused by adherents of interpretative science, assists understanding rather than predicts or prescribes. Relativists may include advocates of phenomenological approaches to nursing science such as Parse (1987) and the founder of the nursing theory of irreducible, unitary human beings, Martha Rogers (1970).

Level two (theory generation level) includes both inductive and deductive approaches to theory generation. Kim states that inductive theory generation requires ' . . . empirically originating generalisations and understanding', whereas deductive theory generation requires ' . . the construction of theoretical systems which are posed for empirical validation' (Kim, 1993). An example of inductive theory generation might be the eliciting of a theory of caring from the lived experiences of nurses in clinical practice. An example of deductive theory could be the testing of a variety of wound healing products on decubitus ulcers in a community nursing setting.

Level three (knowledge type level) includes three kinds of knowledge for nursing: descriptive, explanatory and predictive. Whilst these types of knowledge have a hierarchical relationship, each type is considered by Kim (1993) as self-contained in terms of knowledge generation. Examples may be drawn from the area of nurse–patient interaction. Descriptive theory may emanate from research into the amount and type of interaction within a particular nursing setting. Explanatory theory might arise from an exploration of the effects of the amount and pattern of eye contact on the length of nurse–patient interactions. Predictive theory may be the result of an investigation of relationship between the amount and quality of nurse–patient interaction and the accurate identification of physical and psychosocial needs in terms of patient-defined problems.

The methodology dimension includes the ways scientists deal with the empirical world and comprises: reality orientation level, reality type level and field orientation level (Kim, 1993). In terms of reality orientation level, Kim differentiates *etic*, or constructed and objective representation of the empirical world: an example may be drawn from natural science approaches in medicine upon which the medical model is based; and *emic*, or personal/subjective representation of empirical world by its meanings to the experiencing persons themselves: for example the phenomenological approach to patient experiences. With regard to reality type level, she acknowledges the structure of the empirical world as consisting of qualitative and quantitative aspects. Field orientation level includes experimental design and naturalistic inquiry (Kim, 1993).

Kim (1993) provides a framework derived from this classification system, which identifies 96 possible and appropriate linkages among philosophy, theory and method: for example realistic, deductive and prescriptive knowledge based on etic, quantitative and experimental methods compared to realistic, deductive and explanatory knowledge based on etic, quantitative and naturalistic methods. She further suggests that, although not all linkages are viable for nursing science, scientific pluralism allows generation of contradictory as well as complementary knowledge arising from the different philosophical, theoretical and methodological perspectives taken to study a particular phenomenon. Roy's conceptual model of nursing exemplifies a pluralistic approach to the conceptualization of nursing in her uses of systems theory, theory from the area of psychophysics and concepts from humanism (Roy, 1984). Rival explanations and contradictory prescriptions would require the practitioner to make secondary choices at the practice level, thus the nurse would, via reflective practice, become an integral part of knowledge validation and accumulation.

Kim offers three possible approaches to knowledge validation: an applied research mode; a coherence mode; and a pragmatist mode. Within the applied research mode, knowledge could be verified or validated at the practice level through critical reasoning, personal experiences and application to nursing practice. This could be exemplified within Benner's (1984) notion of the expert practitioner in nursing. Perhaps this also includes the integration of nursing art and science within the experience of the practitioner (Rose and Parker, 1994). Within the coherence mode, nurses' personal orientations would dictate knowledge use in practice. This approach might well facilitate coherence and integration, but could also create undesirable dogmatism arising from habituation and narrowness of vision.

The pragmatist position allows nurses to select knowledge claims and explanations according to their use in solving given problems: testing their usefulness in practice, incorporating into their personal knowledge that which actually works. This allows nurses to focus on final products rather than the processes and philosophies underpinning knowledge development. Kim (1993, p.799) supports scientific pluralism for nursing to allow for '. . . a kaleidoscope of perspectives and use of different lenses for viewing nursing phenomena, both for scientists and practitioners'. She concludes with a word of caution, however, in that this approach requires individual and disciplinary awareness of the meanings of pluralism in terms of knowledge evaluation/cumulation and knowledge utilization in nursing.

According to Johnson (1991), if the science of nursing is to be relevant to the art of nursing, then both art and science must remain connected. In other words, it is not appropriate to pursue theoretical knowledge in its pure form advocated by writers such as Packard and Polifroni (1991), nor would it be fruitful to pursue nursing as an applied science, 'Only if nursing science is conceptualised and pursued as a practical science will the science of nursing be consistently relevant to the art of nursing' (Johnson, 1991). Although acknowledging the group of nurses who have dismissed the entire issue regarding the debate about the nature of nursing science, Johnson suggests that a proper resolution of this issue is necessary for the advancement of nursing as a discipline. The manner in which nursing science is conceptualized will determine the nature of nursing research and the consequential effects of the research on nursing practice. Johnson, like Adam (1987), calls for pluralism of theories in nursing, but suggests that the resultant diversity is not itself an appropriate end for the discipline of nursing. An important assumption underpinning Johnson's work is that explications regarding the nature of nursing science must presuppose the nature of nursing art: nursing science must ultimately serve the art of nursing and not vice versa.

According to Johnson the purpose of basic sciences is the attainment of knowledge for its own sake, whereas the goal of the practical scientist is the development of knowledge that leads to something doable or makeable. If nursing is pursued as basic science, nursing science will be made up entirely of description and explanation. 'Basic scientific knowledge of human phenomena does not provide the nurse with the necessary knowledge to make decisions about the most effective course to follow in meeting a goal' (Johnson, 1991). As a consequence nursing art and science would be left to function and develop in their own separate realms. Johnson urges that nurses should understand the scientific principles that guide their art in order that they can better understand and analyse new situations as they occur and also modify the principles of practice. She criticizes the conceptualization of nursing as an applied science primarily because of the limitations in the development of scientific knowledge directly relevant to the art of nursing; advances in nursing science being limited to the application of existing basic scientific theories. A view of nursing as an application of medical science would restrict nursing to the curing paradigm. The science of nursing would be driven by the advancements of medicine and other disciplines and not by identified needs arising from nursing practice. 'Nursing scientists must be free to develop and test nursing interventions; their endeavours should not be unnecessarily constrained' (Johnson, 1994).

Johnson offers a conceptualization of nursing science as practical science, closely aligning the science of nursing with the art of nursing. The practical sciences are concerned with the doable or makeable, proceed compositively and are applicable to the performance of particular operations. In this way the scientific rules and principles for nursing practice can provide the basis for nursing art. Peplau's (1952) middle range nursing theory drawn from the perspectives of psychoanalytical theory, the principles of social learning, the concept of human motivation and the concept of personality development (Brophy et al, 1994) provided mental health nurses with a clear and meaningful conception of professional practice at a time when medicine dominated the health care field. Although empirically imprecise, Peplau's conceptual framework has been utilized by innumerable researchers and practitioners, with a considerable impact on practice. However well legitimated, scientific knowledge must be complemented by skill and knowledge of the particular situation. 'Nursing is clearly both a science and an art. To disarticulate these two aspects of nursing is to dismember nursing' (Johnson, 1994).

It may be noticeable that the debate on nursing science is repeatedly qualified by pleas to keep integrated the art and science of nursing. Although it would have been possible for the writer to put forward the alternative bias, exhorting nursing science at the expense of nursing art, this sterile objective approach is offensive to someone who loves the practice of nursing. Readers who wish to explore the 'hard' science debate should have little difficulty in accessing the considerable volume of literature that exists. A third strand in the debate is reflection. It may be that reflection-in-action represents a possible mechanism to assist the nurse to integrate practice and theory, science and art.

◆

REFLECTION AND PROFESSIONAL ARTISTRY

Well known and oft quoted work on different ways of knowing (Polyani, 1967; Carper, 1978), together with the writings of philosophers such as Freire (1972), Habermas (1974) and Schotter (1974) on reflection and practice theory, have provided nursing and other scholars with the basis for the existing literature on reflection. It is not my intention to present a review of this work. Chapter 6 provides a full review of this work.

According to Conway (1994) reflection may help nurses to bridge the theory practice gap and provide a process for developing knowledge from practice. Conway accepts Schon's (1987) definitions of reflection as 'his is the only work that presents reflection as occurring in practice, linked to experience and central to the concept of professional artistry' (Conway, 1994). Conway suggests that reflection-in-action occurs in the practice setting; requires practitioners to think on their feet; involves a type of action research; cannot be taught, but coaching can promote its development; can be seen in the performance of practitioner who demonstrates 'professional artistry' and can be used as a paradigm for learning from practice. Conway discusses the limitations of the technical rationality paradigm and concludes that by itself it is inadequate for nursing. She advocates the development of artistry in nursing to facilitate the acquisition of knowledge from practice. 'Through the development of professional artistry the practitioner is able not only to deal with manageable problems that lend themselves to solutions through the application of research-based theory, but also to deal with the often messy problems of daily nursing practice' (Conway, 1994). This is clearly linked to Schon's (1987) description of the swampy lowland, where messy, confusing problems defy technical solution. In an important statement Schon encapsulates a compelling argument for the application of reflection-in-action through professional artistry: 'The irony of the situation is that the problems of the high ground tend to be relatively unimportant to individuals or society at large . . . while in the swamp lie the problems of greatest human concern' (Conway, 1994). By the high ground Schon is referring to scientific knowledge from the rationalistic paradigm.

It appears to me that this call for professional artistry is compelling. In an era where nursing is becoming increasingly accepted as a scientific discipline, where nurses are increasingly regarded as highly educated professionals, there seems to me to be a danger of professional distancing and a reduction in the perceived importance of caring in nursing practice. As scientific knowledge is viewed as rigorous, so too can professional artistry be rigorous in terms of its delivery in a milieu which demands the use of critical evaluation of nursing practice within a structure of clinical supervision. Developing knowledge through reflection-in-action is more likely to incorporate nursing's essential caring and humanistic approaches to people and their needs. Conway (1994) further suggests that there are additional potentialities for reflection-in-action as a means of developing unique nursing knowledge.

'Reflection-in-action, as demonstrated in the professional artistry of expert practitioners, is a process in which the art of the practitioner fuses with a form of action research to produce a science of practice. If this process is reflected on, it is possible for the knowledge that is found in practical nursing knowledge to be identified and developed into theories, which in turn can guide and inform practice' (Conway, 1994).

Intuitively this sounds feasible and admirable, but there remain many obstacles to be overcome, not the least of which is the difficulty, pointed out by Schon (1987), of the practitioners who are unable to articulate the knowledge that they use. What we need are practitioners who are able and willing to examine their work in critical ways and scholars and researchers who are able to develop nursing's knowledge base in this way. It seems to me that what is required are practitioners who are also scholars and researchers. Looking at the nature of nursing academia and practice, not only in the United Kingdom, but also in the United States, Canada and Australia, we still have some way to go to achieve this goal. In the United Kingdom we have a national health service where clinical supervision is being introduced across all nursing specialisms (DoH, 1994). The haphazard implementation in practice appears to match the blanket approach through which the nursing process was forced onto nurses in the late 1970s. This mirrors the less than critical acceptance of reflection in Project 2000 curricula in the late 1980s (Rich and Parker, 1995). As a result of reflecting in the classroom we have students who are experiencing the increasing divide between academia and practice. Unskilled facilitation of reflection-on-action tends to focus on the negative, particularly in a situation where anxiety levels are high. This may ultimately result in hostility between the lecturers and practitioners who facilitate reflection-on-action with students in an attempt to nurture their ability to reflect-in-action.

Newell (1992) notes the practical difficulties associated with reflection, those related to the mediating effects of memory and anxiety. He further identifies general problems such as lack of conceptual clarity and lack of evaluative studies (Newell, 1994). He suggests that we could argue that 'reflection is a creative art, like painting or music, and that, as such, it confers benefits which are intrinsic to the pursuit of reflection and are, in consequence, not amenable to empirical support or refutation' (Newell, 1994). This is certainly supported by many of the writers introduced in this chapter and elsewhere. It is also logical that certain personal types of reflection are indeed not able to be transformed into scientific data by virtue of their tacit nature. Subjective reflection, however critical, is not enough; these beliefs are insufficient justification for the current widespread adoption of reflection. Newell questions whether the claims made for reflection are empirical ones; if reflection changes practice, then it should be possible, and essential, for professionals to define what constitutes reflection in a way that allows its efficacy to be tested in terms of outcomes for patients and nurses. Perhaps reflective practitioners, not ivory tower academics, may be the nurses who are able to take forward the profession of nursing into the 21st century.

In summary, this chapter has outlined the debate regarding art and science in nursing. It has reviewed the literature behind this debate, and has introduced ideas, such as caring, intuition, morality and reflection. These form threads throughout the book, and are the basis of subsequent chapters.

Conversation

CHAPTER 2   *One of the things I noticed is the way your use of language changed from the language of the artist, descriptive and personal, to the language of the scientist, inaccessible to the average nurse and patient, and impersonal.*

CHAPTER 1   *Yes, this was deliberate, to emphasize that the different perspectives are not only in content but in presentation as well.*

CHAPTER 2   *It's like opposite faces of the cube. When one is visible, the other is in shadow. I found the jargon in the section on science heavy going, but I see it would be impossible to discuss science using the language of art.*

CHAPTER 1   *Yes, Chapter 7 has more to say about this. It seems to me that I have presented the historical and current position of art and science in nursing. I have shown how art and science are used as metaphors for nursing, that is, nursing is like art, and like science.*

CHAPTER 2   *I want to go a stage further. I want to demonstrate that nursing is art, not just like art, and uses science and technology in the creative process. . . .*

SCIENCE AND TECHNOLOGY: TOOLS IN THE CREATION OF NURSING

Pat Rose

Nursing as an art and a science is an issue which has exercised the minds of nurses since Florence Nightingale first suggested that it is both, a claim still made today (UKCC, 1992a). The history and nature of this debate has been fully explored in the previous chapter. However, whilst hesitating to add to what some may view as a subject which has been done to death, I believe that the necessity for clarity on the issue is perhaps never more urgent than today. Nursing is seeking to establish itself as an academic discipline and claim a knowledge base commensurate with its situation within the higher education institutions where knowledge has traditionally been divided into the arts and the sciences. Nurses are increasingly seeking to study nursing as opposed to related disciplines (Watson, 1981) and as higher awards are being offered in the study of nursing the debate becomes more pragmatic as the virtues of, for example, a Masters in Nursing (MN), as opposed to MSc in Nursing, or indeed MA in Nursing, are discussed.

The purpose of this chapter is to propose a new way of looking at the issue. I will explore the notion that it is nursing itself which is a work of art, created by the nurse as the artist, using science and technology as the tools, for patients as the audience. Thus this chapter will examine the nature of art, the use of science and technology in nursing, and the roles of the nurse and patient with these in mind.

Examples will be drawn upon from literature and research, and will be illustrated by reflection on my own experiences as a nurse and a patient.

In the development of nursing theory there has been a move from logical positivism towards the interpretive and critical sciences. In describing the early stages of theory development in nursing, Cull-Wilby and Pepin (1987) suggest that, although nursing is a profession of human interaction, caring and nurturing, within a social context, it has attempted to adhere to describing its world of human interaction by the positivist scientific methods which were designed to explain phenomena of the physical world. Thus nursing, they argue, has partly lost sight of the importance of the art of nursing. They suggest, however, that the emphasis of nursing research has now gone full circle and returned to Nightingale's emphasis on the person and the environment.

Smith (1981) suggests that, although not lost, the art of nursing has been justified entirely in terms of compassion, humanity, ideals of service, and so on. He goes on to suggest that if the art of nursing is to be rationally justified, it must rest on a scientific basis. He asserts that nursing is the art of applying nursing science; however, in examining nursing as an art I believe that one must differentiate between 'the art of nursing' and 'nursing as an art form'. The art of nursing may be the process by which nursing as an art form emerges, but it could equally well be the process by which nursing as a science is expressed. Whilst it may be possible to explore this process from a scientific basis, the exploration of nursing art must be rooted in the philosophy and theory of art.

In the previous chapter, David Parker introduced the work of Johnson (1994), who conducted a study to explore opinion regarding the art of nursing. She analysed the works of 41 authors and identified five separate senses of nursing art (Table 2.1).

It is interesting to note that she did not find any use of nursing art in the sense of nursing being an art form, or indeed of the notion of creativity. There are examples in the literature in which art such as weaving (Gendron, 1994) and dance (Parse, 1992a) have been used as metaphors for nursing. What seems to be missing is any exploration of what exactly is the work of art created in nursing, if any, and, based on the assumption that art needs an audience, who its audience is.

◆ Table 2.1	**Five Senses of Nursing Art (Johnson, 1994).**	
	Sense of 'nursing art'	**Nursing art characterized by:**
	Ability to grasp meaning in patient encounters	Perceptual capacity outside of intellect Immediacy, knowing what to do as situations arise Tacit knowledge, understanding that defies complete or accurate description
	Ability to establish a meaningful connection with the patient	Being expressed in action not words Expressive of emotions and sentiments, e.g. compassion, caring Occurring in relation to others as equals Authenticity, the nurse is not just acting a role, and does not mask her feelings
	Ability to perform nursing activities skilfully	Behavioural ability Skilful performance learned by practice Being judged by descriptors such as adroitness, coordination, flow of movement, manual dexterity, efficiency
	Ability to determine rationally an appropriate course of nursing action	Being practical in nature Resting on an underlying theoretical discipline The nurse understanding the situation and knowing what action is appropriate, applying scientific theory Logical reasoning Being goal-led and judged against standards
	Ability to conduct one's nursing practice morally	Making moral choices in performance of care Skill and knowledge not being enough Commitment to practice competently A moral nature in the nurse, proper motivation

◆

NURSING AND THE THEORY OF ART

My starting point in exploring some of these issues is to examine the ideas addressed within the philosophy and theory of art. To do this it is important to hold in abeyance the assumptions of science, and embrace the world-view of the artist. A dictionary definition of art states that it is both a human creative skill or its application (*Concise Oxford Dictionary*, 1991). It is argued that art is, things acquired or produced by craft or skill (Rose and Parker, 1994), and is learned rather than taught by nature or instinct; thus to walk is natural, to dance is art (Crystal, 1990). Both these ideas are apparent in nursing. First, nursing occurs as a result of human endeavour, it is not a natural phenomenon; and secondly nursing is learned as opposed to instinctual. However this is not enough to say that therefore nursing is art.

Another way of defining art is to say that it is something that not only fulfils the description above, but also that it is aesthetically pleasing, or beautiful. Harrison-Barbet (1990) poses the question of whether there are criteria that must be fulfilled for something to be considered aesthetically pleasing, or whether it is simply it a matter of subjective opinion. He suggested a comparison between the music of a pop group and that of Beethoven, or romantic fiction compared to the works of Tolstoy, and asked which could be considered art, or whether they are all art carrying varying degrees of artistic value. In discussing aesthetic beauty in art the concept of form is important. Form is the arrangement of elements to create a complex unity which arouses strong feelings in the observer. For example, in painting, the elements are colours and shapes, in music they are the musical notes and rhythms, and in ballet the movements of the dancers choreographed to create the whole. In nursing the elements could be those concepts identified by theorists and arranged to create a nursing model or conceptual framework, for example the concepts of universal self-care requisites, self-care deficit, and so on used by Orem (1985). However, patients may not find a conceptual framework aesthetically pleasing and I will suggest that the elements in nursing are all those activities which make up the role of the nurse, including complex technical skills, meeting hygiene needs, listening, teaching and so on, arranged to create a whole which is pleasing to the patient.

Langer (1957), however, suggested that to define art in terms of beauty is not possible because of the problem that what is considered beautiful in one era, or by one section of society, is considered ugly by another. She went on to suggest, however, that it is possible to define art for all time in all contexts, as apparent forms, that is those created by human skill rather than occurring naturally, which are expressive of human feeling, and which were created for that purpose. Thus she argued that crafts which are sometimes called arts, such as the art of cooking, are not art because though the purpose may be to evoke feeling, it is not to express feeling. She went on to suggest that a large part of the world's art was not made with the conscious intention of creating art, but with the intention of making, or performing, or otherwise articulating some important human emotion. For example religious artefacts were often made with the intention of expressing human wonder, awe, or praise of a god or goddess, and therefore have become labelled as works of art. If one subscribes to this view the question is whether nursing expresses some human emotion, regardless of intention. I suggest that it does, that nursing is the expression of emotions such as caring, and compassion, and optimism.

Sheppard (1987) suggests that expression is, actually, not a definition of art, but one opinion as to its purpose, and that it is wrong to suggest that the purpose of all art is expression. Expression, as a purpose of art, involves the communication of emotions with the aim of evoking a response. For example, the artist might communicate love by writing a poem, power by composing a symphony, shock and confusion through a cubist painting, or disgust through a pickled sheep. In nursing, the emotions a nurse might wish to communicate include calmness, hope, and confidence. The difficulty with this view of art is that individuals have different emotional responses to the same stimuli as evident in the comments of different art critics regarding the same piece of work. So, in nursing, a nurse might make a flippant remark which would communicate the humour of a situation to one audience but might express something entirely different to another. An example of this happened to me during a hospital admission. At the time I had suffered from a painful condition for over two years and medical intervention had been unsuccessful. During that time I had gradually reduced the physical activity I undertook as I found exercise exacerbated the pain. Always a fat person, I became even fatter. Eventually it was decided that abdominal surgery to have the diseased organ removed was the appropriate course of action. I had returned from theatre at about 1 pm and it was now about 8 pm. My IVI had tissued and a doctor had come to re-site it. A nurse was there to re-connect the giving set once the cannula had been inserted, but also, I assume, to create an environment of care for me.

I had no fear of the cannulation. I knew what to expect, and nothing could compare to the pain I had felt when the patient-controlled analgesia had failed due to the tissued drip. I was very relaxed, having had intra-muscular pain relief. I felt extremely safe and all my care to date had been exemplary. I was finding the whole process of being a patient very interesting having been a nurse for so long.

The doctor searched both my hands and arms, looking for a vein to cannulate. He peered closely at the back of my left hand, then my forearm above the wrist. He reached across the bed for my right arm. The hand and wrist were swollen from the tissued infusion. He looked at my elbow. Rejecting that arm he returned to my left hand, and asked the nurse to squeeze my forearm. Still no vein became visible but he thought he felt a vein and inserted the needle. It failed. As he moved to the elbow of that arm the nurse said, 'Next time you come to hospital for surgery you will have to do six months weight training before you come, then you'll have veins like Schwarzenegger'. I dissolved into tears.

It is recognized that humour is a useful tool in the nursing repertoire. It can be used to break down barriers, diffuse an emotionally charged atmosphere, establish rapport, reassure, and convey information (Harries, 1995). However, as with any tool, if humour is not used knowledgeably, and with sensitivity to the context, it can be destructive. When the nurse made her humorous comment to me, I felt overwhelmed with grief. I suddenly felt acutely the loss of the exercise I used to enjoy, and realized the impact the protracted illness had had on my life. I pictured my garden, how its beauty had degenerated into a complete mess as I had gradually done less and less in it. I remembered my early morning Sunday swim, and breakfast with friends each week, friends I rarely saw now as I could no longer participate in the activity that had brought us together. The loss was suddenly intolerable. Far from injecting humour to relieve tension, the nurse, by the flippant remark, had expressed to me total insensitivity. I was the wrong audience to enjoy the humour. If the nurse had been knowledgeable about me and my history, and sensitive to my feelings, she would not have made this remark.

Sheppard (1987) moves on from the idea of the purpose of art as being expression, to a discussion of its purpose of arousing aesthetic emotion or feeling. This differs from expression as the aim here is to actually arouse feeling in others not simply express it. The post-modernist view is that if something someone has created, whatever it is, arouses any strong feeling then this is art. A dead sheep in formaldehyde, a heap of tyres, or a discordant sonata would therefore be art because it has achieved the purpose of arousing strong feelings. Likewise, while my IVI was being sited, the remark by the nurse resulted in strong feelings being aroused in me. She did not know what type of feeling her remark would arouse; she had probably used that particular line with others in the past with laughter resulting. However, that the remark did raise strong feelings in me, therefore, could be classed as art according to this viewpoint.

As well as illustrating different people's responses to well-intentioned nursing activity the incident of the flippant remark raises the issue of morality in nursing. It does not really matter if I do not like the music of a particular composer, I can choose what music to listen to. However, it does matter if, as a patient, I am exposed to nursing care which I do not choose, because I simply find it displeasing to me, or it may actually harm me. Nurses are required not to do things which are detrimental to patients, but to promote their well-being (UKCC, 1992a), and must therefore hone their art to individual patients, a point I will return to later in discussing nursing care in relation to human uniqueness.

It could be argued that art is something people go to see, or hear, or read, as an audience, because they expect to find it pleasing or at least interesting. In thinking of art in its usual conceptions, painting, music, drama, and so on, one imagines the audience choosing what to attend, buying a ticket, and turning up on the day. The patient as audience of nursing art, however, does not choose to be in the position to require nursing, does not choose what to view, and is either instructed what day to turn up, or in the case of emergencies, is simply taken to the show.

Rafferty (1987) suggests that one of the characteristics of art is that it occurs in abnormal settings, such as a gallery or theatre, not in places where people spend their time on a day to day basis. A hospital, in this context, is an abnormal place. However it is not entirely true to say that art occurs in abnormal places. We pass art, in the form of architecture, every day as we walk through the streets of the city, town or village in which we live. We use, or see, art in our daily activities, on the cover of a book, in the designs of our curtains and in the random background music we hear on the radio. We do not choose as audience, when and where we will see or hear this art, it is part of our everyday life. Thus I would argue that art is an unusual occurrence, created for the expression and eliciting of emotion, in any setting. Often, however we pass by that art, and far from perceiving its artistic merit we do not ever notice it is there. Nursing, such as being given sometimes intimate care, by a stranger, often in the presence of other strangers, is not a usual occurrence. Nor indeed is the doctor's surgery, or hospital ward, a usual setting. Many people experience nursing, but, as with other forms of art, its artistic value passes them by.

The requirement that art needs an audience may not be true. Just as with other forms of art, not everyone who encounters nursing will give it more than passing recognition. Mitchell (1992) discusses the issue of perceiving art, in relation to those with sensory loss. For example those with hearing loss can 'hear' music through vibrations from the floor, and those with visual loss 'see' a painting through a detailed aural description. She adds that the art experienced by these people is not the same as the art experienced by someone without the sensory loss. Thus, the perception of nursing art may depend on the 'receptors' used by the patient. If the patient is unable to use their sense of humour they will not perceive an attempt by the nurse to lighten a situation, as funny. The art this patient perceives will be a different art. However, the person with hearing or visual loss experiences emotional effect despite what they perceive being different to that which was intended, so the humorous remark by a nurse elicits a different emotion than was intended, thus it remains art. The problem with this however, as discussed earlier, is that it is not acceptable for a nurse to expose the patient to art which may cause harm.

Another theory of the purpose of art which Sheppard (1987) explores is that of imitation, or in its widest sense, representation. This is the idea that art seeks to provide a bridge between eternal ideas, such as love or beauty, and the way in which they are sensed by individuals, by expressing them in a perceivable form such as poetry or music. Perhaps, in relation to this, nursing is aiming to bridge the gap between the idea of health, and the perception of being healthy. The nurse, through a knowledge of physical, behavioural and social sciences, has an idea of health for an individual. This, combined with the individual's own view of health, becomes the goal for care. In the delivery of care, the nurse carries out those activities the person is unable to do for themselves, and teaches and supports the patient in those activities which they can or wish to do. Thus, whilst the patient is not self-caring, there is an imitation of health as the nurse builds the bridge between the idea and the reality.

Nursing as art then, provides an imitation of health to the patient who has a health deficit. In the role of health promoter too nurses may be representing health to the patient. For example when teaching sexual health to school children, the nurse offers them the ideal, the means to achieve it, and hopefully the motivation to do so. Again a bridge is built between the idea of being sexually healthy, and the perception of it for school children.

The ideas explored so far have examined the notion of nursing as art in relation to some of the concepts and ideas arising within the philosophy and theory of art. Illustrative examples from nursing have been drawn on to support the idea that nursing is an art form. However it is important not merely to look for individual ideas in separate incidents but also to examine a nursing encounter to see how far all the ideas are represented within it. For this I will, using reflective processes, analyse an incident which occurred in my own practice as a children's nurse.

The setting was a children's ward where I was to care for a baby, whom I will call Joe, for the afternoon and evening. Joe was 13 months old. During the course of the morning he had been transferred from another hospital. On arrival he had undergone a lumbar puncture and intravenous cannulation. He was refusing fluids orally, had a high pyrexia, and was miserable and lethargic. The cause of his condition remained a mystery. Using the reflective process I will focus on my first encounter with Joe and his mother.

Put simply the incident was the occasion when I introduced myself to Joe's mother, explained what I intended to do and lifted the cot-side to gain access to the baby. My reflective observations of what happened and how I felt were as follows.

As I entered Joe's room his mother stood to greet me. Joe lay sprawled across his cot, naked apart from a nappy, sound asleep. I knew he was sleeping, not unconscious, by his colour, the rhythm of his breathing, and his posture which indicated good muscle tone. I introduced myself to Joe's mother and explained that I would be helping her to care for Joe for the next eight hours. She described what they had been through during the course of the morning. In her body was a tension, born of anxiety, and in her eyes an appeal which said to me, 'Please don't hurt my baby any more.' I explained that I must check Joe's temperature.

I moved to the cot and, standing on one leg to release the catch with my other knee, I took the weight of the heavy metal bars in both hands to lift the cot-side down. To prevent the catch clanking back as I lifted the bars from their cradle, I continued to support it with my knee, thus completing the manoeuvre balancing on one leg. Gently I eased down the catch, then lowered the cot-side silently. I was aware of Joe's mother at my side with hands poised to catch the bars should I falter, but my eyes remained on the sleeping baby, knowing I would have to act quickly if he rolled.

As I moved my body to protect the sleeping child, vulnerable now without the cot-side, I looked across at his mother. We made eye contact and in that moment I knew she trusted me. I knew it by the almost imperceptible relaxation of her body, by the easing of her facial muscles, and by the message of her eyes giving me permission to touch her son.

By my simple act of lowering a cot-side without disturbing her baby, a mother felt able to entrust to me the well-being, potentially the life, of her child. Thus began a partnership of care for the precious baby.

What was I thinking and feeling through this interaction? First, as I entered the room I knew I must gain the mother's confidence quickly. Joe would need my attention for at least ten minutes of each hour to check his vital signs and neurological status, and monitor his fluid balance. In addition his mother would need care as she managed her own distress, and comforted her baby and encouraged him to drink.

As I lifted the cot-side I was determined that the baby would not wake. I felt confident of achieving this. I had carried out the manoeuvre many times before. Nevertheless, I was relieved when it was successfully completed. Finally, when I looked into the eyes of the mother and knew she trusted me I felt a pride, both in myself, and in my profession. I was keenly aware of the responsibility I now carried, but felt very privileged that a mother could allow me to share in the care of her sick child.

In examining the incident in relation to the theory of art I began by considering expression. It seemed clear that the action of lowering a cot-side quietly so as not to wake a baby, was an expression of caring for them, or to use Benner and Wrubel's (1989) definition, an expression of the fact that they *mattered* to me. The visible relaxation of the mother indicated that my action had had an impact on her, the emotion I believed I elicited was trust. My subsequent interactions with this mother confirmed that view. For example, later in the afternoon, when Joe was awake, she asked me to sit with him while she went to get herself a cup of tea. Thus I believe that in this act of nursing there was intention to express feeling, as well as response elicited from the audience.

From here I moved on to consider representation. If this nursing action expresses caring, could it be that it is a representation of the caring that an individual would receive from those closest to them if they had the knowledge and ability to provide that care. I could never be Joe's mother but my care could represent that which she would give but in a situation where her care was limited by lack of knowledge of the care and management a sick baby needs. Or perhaps the nursing action was an imitation of the mother's care; a copy. Within the Partnership Model for nursing (Casey, 1988), one of the tenets of children's nursing is family-centred care. This is built on the idea that children, sick or well, are best cared for by their own family. The role of the nurse is to provide, or teach the family, the care the child needs associated with the medical diagnosis, treatment or other health problems, that the family are unable to give due to their lack of knowledge and skills. By representing the family, the idea of family care, which underpins the model, is thus presented by the nurse in a form which is perceivable to the family.

In terms of form, the use of the elements in nursing, this encounter used the following elements:

1. Establishing a relationship with the patients by introducing myself and giving an explanation of my role.
2. Observation, of mother and child.
3. Interpretation of data obtained by observation of the baby, and his mother, and based on knowledge of

physiology, psychology, normal child development, and on intuition, my own tacit knowledge.

4. Knowledge of equipment, the cot.
5. Manual dexterity, in quietly lifting the cot side.
6. Body language and gesture, in moving to protect the baby from rolling, and making eye contact with the mother.
7. Ethical knowledge, knowing what was the right thing to do in the unique circumstances.

All these elements were combined to create a unique whole within this unique encounter. In this case that which was created was tangible, it was a relationship of trust between Joe's mother and myself. In other nursing situations the mix of these, and other elements, such as complex medical technology, counselling skills, teaching skills and all the other aspects of nursing practice, might be combined to create another unique incident of nursing. This I contend is nursing as art.

This reflection on practice has demonstrated that the concepts of art are indeed present in nursing. Thus having examined the possibility of nursing as an art form, it is necessary to return to science and technology, both of which undoubtedly have an important role within the discipline of nursing. I will argue however that this role is not in defining what nursing is but in providing the tools with which the nurse, as artist, creates nursing.

♦

SCIENCE AND TECHNOLOGY IN NURSING PRACTICE

The word 'science' is rooted in the Latin 'scientia' meaning knowledge. In its pure sense therefore, science does not assume the nature of reality, only that it is knowable. Powers and Knapp (1990) maintain this pure view of science in defining it as an activity combining research (the advancement of knowledge), with theory (the explanation of knowledge). However, Polit and Hungler (1993) suggest that science is the most sophisticated method of acquiring knowledge that humans have developed, and that in problem solving, although fallible, is more reliable than tradition, authority, experience, or trial and error. Scientific inquiry is dependent on rigorous data collection, analysis and interpretation and its values are scepticism, doubt, objectivity and detachment (Peplau, 1988). Reed and Procter (1993) suggest that, because of these values, science is viewed as a superior form of knowledge, which carries high academic status. It is this view that led to an emphasis on scientific research in nursing and the emergence of the term 'nursing science' in the 1950s (Carper, 1978).

Carper (1978) suggested that the highly integrated, abstract and systematic explanations are the 'ideal form' of science, that is the hypothetical model against which reality is measured, to which nursing aspires, but which had not yet been reached in what was a relatively new discipline. This quest for nursing science, and the contribution it has made to nursing must not be under-emphasized and its momentum is not subsiding. Thus it is relevant here to review briefly the paradigms or world-views of the nature of reality, as this contributes to the suggestion that nursing is an art form which uses science and technology as its tools.

Rationalistic enquiry is based on the assumption that there is an objective reality, outside human perception, which can be explored and known through the processes of logical thinking, and can lead to facts or positive certainties; hence the term positivism often used as a synonym for rationalistic science.

Positivism was a term coined by the philosopher Auguste Comte (1798–1857) who proposed that all aspects of the world could be reduced to observable phenomena from which theory could be induced and tested, resulting in certain, or positive, knowledge. It became the predominant force in scientific enquiry and remains a strong influence to this day.

Positivism is sometimes termed the 'received view' because it is dependent on data received by the senses. According to Watson (1981) the received view is characterized by reductionism, quantifiability, objectivity, and the possibility of operationalization. In nursing, this approach is useful in generating knowledge related to biological needs, and effects of physical care. For example, measurement of vital signs and neurological status, issues related to dietary needs, pressure area management, and fluid balance. Those espousing this view of reality would also suggest that people have predictable responses to stimuli such as stress, loss and hospitalization, and that social groups, such as social classes, women and youth have a predictable range of characteristics. As a discipline involved in all aspects of human experience, nursing has been profoundly influenced by rationalistic science. Indeed the very process of nursing, the systematic collection of data, diagnosis of nursing problems, goal setting, care planning and delivery and finally measurement of outcomes has been labelled a scientific approach (Marriner, 1975).

The nursing process seems to rest comfortably on the positivist nursing cube face, based on the assumption that there is an objective reality which can be established by systematic, rationalistic enquiry. Barnum (1994) goes as far as to suggest that the greatest appeal of the nursing process is in its offer of a system of uniform practice, and the possibility of applying quantitative measures. She adds that the commitment to rationalistic research by nurses may account for the popularity of the nursing process.

Concurrent with the development of a systematic approach to nursing care has been the development of ever more sophisticated tools to predict, measure and quantify the outcomes of care. One of the earliest tools in prevention of pressure sores was the Norton pressure area risk score (Norton et al, 1962), and other more sophisticated tools have been developed since (Warterlow, 1985; Bergstrom et al, 1987), and culminated in the publication of national clinical guidelines, developed using scientific processes (Dealey, 1996). Nurses have also adopted and further developed tools originating in medicine such as the Glasgow coma scale (Teasdale and Jennett, 1974) which has been developed into the Neurological Assessment Instrument (Way and Segatore, 1994). Using tools such as these, assessment data are collected and analysed. In its most sophisticated form specific combinations of data will lead to a specific nursing diagnosis being made (Kim et al, 1993), though in Britain this process is not well established and nurses tend, rather, to synthesize a nursing problem following data collection and analysis.

Care planning ideally involves prescribing a package of care, which research has demonstrated will achieve the desired outcome. For example, when a child has a high temperature, the goal is that the temperature will be normal and a prescribed care protocol, based in research, is to reduce clothing, tepid sponge and give prescribed paracetamol (Kinmouth, 1992). The use of care protocols has developed into a system now known as 'managed care', in which a care map, or multidisciplinary action plan, is established, based on the needs of people with particular medical diagnoses (Laxade and Hale, 1995).

Managed care is, however, in its infancy (Hale, 1995) and in reality, prescribed care often has more to do with tradition and ward routine than research. One of the criticisms of managed care is that there is a risk that individualized care, so highly prized by nurses that it is enshrined within ethical principles within which we practice (UKCC, 1992a), may become lost (Laxade and Hale, 1995). There is perhaps some value in the ritual of tradition and ward routine. It presents opportunities for the nurse to find out more about the patient, and thus reduces the risk of harm to the patient, such as the case described earlier when a nurse made an inappropriate attempt at humour. Ritual nursing actions, though not therapeutic in themselves, create an environment, and relationships, in which rational nursing activities can take place. The use of care and treatment based on tradition is, of course, not unique to nursing. Much of medical practice, although making scientific claims, has not been tested using rationalistic methods, and doctors base their decisions on what they call their 'clinical judgement' (Hammond, 1994; Maynard, 1994).

During care delivery, data are collected to measure movement towards the goal and at the stated time a summative evaluation is made of achievement of the desired outcome. In keeping with the view that rationalistic science holds supremacy over other forms of knowledge, there has been increasing pressure on nurses to demonstrate a measurable impact on patients as a result of care given. This has led to a new label, 'outcome research', to describe the emergent literature on the subject (Bond and Thomas, 1991; Douglas and Robb, 1995; Griffiths, 1995; Newens, 1995). This drive towards rationalistic, objective, predictable nursing practice has led to the need for accurate reliable tools for assessment and care delivery. This, in turn, has led to the development of more and more advanced technology for use in nursing practice.

The term technology is used by nurses to describe a wide range of equipment and techniques including drugs, mechanical and electronic devices, and the medical and surgical techniques which use them, as well as support systems such as those for computerized information (Wichowski, 1994). Allan and Hall (1988) suggest that technology relies on, and reinforces, Cartesian dualism in which the mind and body are viewed as separate entities, and is focused in the physical body.

The use of technology is not new in the care of the sick. Bullough and Bullough (1979) describe the use of moulded splints, made from linen impregnated with glue and plaster,

in ancient Egypt. However, medical – and hence nursing –
technology proliferated as the industrial revolution advanced.
Early technological tools to aid assessment include the glass
and mercury thermometer, and the stethoscope. The
thermometer has evolved to become an electronic device in
which sensors may be attached to various parts of the body,
and probes inserted into orifices including the mouth, rectum
and ear. Likewise the simple stethoscope, used to assess the
sound of the heart is giving way to the ECG monitor which
provides a picture of the electrical impulses, or even to
scanners which can actually view the heart in action.

In the delivery of care, nursing technology includes
pressure-relieving beds, mechanical hoists for lifting and
moving patients, and a wide range of devices to aid
continence. Technology to provide treatment, as opposed to
assisting assessment or care, has also been developed. Hill
and Summers (1994) describe the evolution of the modern
ventilator from heart–lung machines used to support the
victims of poliomyelitis, to the extracorporeal membrane
oxygenator which can bypass the lungs altogether. In almost
all aspects of care, technology plays a major part, and the
greater the use of technology the higher the status of the
specialism concerned.

In its development technology is rooted in rationalistic
science. Based on powerful microcomputers, technological
monitoring devices are designed to make reliable responses
to stimuli, and are thus viewed as more accurate than human
assessment. For example, a thermometer will give a more
accurate measure of a persons temperature than will a hand
on a fevered brow. In care delivery technology is viewed as
more efficient and effective. For example a mechanical
pressure-relieving bed will provide more regular and
consistent pressure changes than two-hourly turns on a
standard mattress. Thus in assessment and delivery of
nursing care the use of technology means that an accurate
account of a persons physical condition can be made, and
the care they have received can be accurately documented.
Outcomes can then be clearly measured and attributed to
the care given. In this way a rational and objective
assessment of progress can be made.

Martin (1990, p.43) suggests that a computer is a model
of rationality which 'works by an infallible process of cause
and effect' but which, by the same token is 'also the very
model of mindless obedience'. It is this mindlessness of
technology which has led some nurses to question its

supremacy in the care of the sick. The ways in which the view of reality as objective and predictable, are influencing nursing as described above, clearly have a value in nursing practice. They have, however, led to the view that nursing itself is a science, rather than simply acknowledging that nursing uses science and technology within its practice. Radcliffe (1995), unimpressed by this view, questions why nursing should wish to be considered a science at all. He dismisses as nonsense, the notion that the science alone has the ability to validate progressive or new ideas. He argues that some aspects of nursing are spontaneous and creative and deal with the experiences and emotions of patients. Watson (1981) suggests that in the quest for science, the characteristics opposing those of positivism, such as subjectivity, quality, emotion, and holism, have become submerged by this emphasis on rationalism. However it is these characteristics which underpin human uniqueness.

As objective realities, human beings usually have physiological senses including sight, hearing, touch, taste, and smell. Unique to individuals, however, are the preferences expressed when using those senses. Using sight, that which is aesthetically pleasing art to one person is seen as a meaningless jumble of colours to another. One person will enjoy choral music whilst another prefers heavy metal. In relation to touch we differ as to which parts of our bodies give us pleasure when touched, and in what we perceive as painful. Our differing food preferences suggest differing perceptions of taste and choices of perfume demonstrate differences in the sense of smell.

In emotional responses too, human uniqueness is evident. Whilst one will laugh at a joke another will find it distasteful. Some enjoy practical jokes and teasing whereas this embarrasses others acutely. Some cry easily at a 'weepy movie' whilst others do not. In response to major disasters some will contribute financially to an appeal for help, others will rush off to the country concerned, or establish an aid organization, whilst many show passing concern only, or indeed voyeurism. In sexual responses one person may be attracted to someone of the same sex and others find the opposite sex attractive.

◆

**THE UNDER-
STANDING OF
HUMAN
UNIQUENESS
IN NURSING**

This recognition of human uniqueness in nursing was like turning the cube to reveal another face, and led to the emergence of naturalistic science as a method of enquiry. Naturalistic science developed as a reaction against positivism. Its objective is to seek knowledge of the underlying meaning of phenomena, or discover the experience of them, as perceived by the individuals or groups involved. It is based on the assumption that there is no reality outside human perception and that as the nature of human experience is subjective, and unique to each individual so the understanding of it must be likewise. Hence the term naturalistic to describe this type of science. Thus reductionist methodology is replaced by phenomenology, ethnomethodology and other humanistic approaches. Nevertheless the rigorous data collection and analysis which are part of the philosophical base of science are retained, thus justifying the inclusion of this type of enquiry under the umbrella of science. In nursing this approach can be used to gain a knowledge of the experience of phenomena for patients, for example, what it is like to have pain, or limited mobility.

Munhall (1993) suggests that this quest to describe experiences in a naturalistic way is the antecedent to rationalistic enquiry, and therefore essential to it. She describes the search for knowledge as a non-linear schema, which she depicts as a spiral. At the centre is discovery of a phenomenon. The spiral then moves through description of that phenomenon, to theory, hypothesis and validation. At this stage a nuance or small variation may be identified and the processes of description, theory development, and testing resume. This cyclical continuum demonstrates how one phenomenon can have multiple, related, nuances all of which lend themselves to research. However, as each phenomenon and nuance must first be described, as it appears in the experience of people, Munhall (1993) calls this type of enquiry first-order activity. The importance of this type of research in nursing becomes apparent as the basic requirements of the Code of Professional Conduct (UKCC, 1992a) are reviewed. Nurses are required to recognize and respect the uniqueness of individual patients and clients and in order to do this must understand that uniqueness. By exploring phenomena, and their variations in the lives of individuals, the uniqueness of each is acknowledged.

In discussing phenomenological philosophy as a way of

exploring individual experiences, Husserl (1970) introduces the idea of the intersubjective constitution of the world. He contended that the basic character of being is consciousness, but that it is not possible to be conscious without being conscious of something. This characteristic of consciousness, being conscious of, he called intentionality. This phenomenon of intentionality means that the object of consciousness becomes the reality of the person concerned. Thus, if I am thinking of a cream cake, that cake is a reality for me. Husserl goes on to suggest that where two people, both of whom have intentionality, interrelate and bring their realities together a new reality is constituted. In thinking of a cream cake, my reality is a vanilla slice. However, I tell a friend that I really fancy a cream cake and her mind automatically turns towards a chocolate eclair. As soon as the two of us tell each other the type of cream cake we would like we both then recognize a new reality: that there is more than one type of cream cake. Through intersubjective constitution of the world a new meaning of the idea of cream cake is synthesized.

In phenomenological research the quest is to seek the meaning of the world in the experience of the individual concerned. For example in exploring the meaning of cream cakes the phenomenologist would ask the subjects 'what is your experience of cream cakes?' The importance of understanding peoples' reality can be illustrated by imagining that I go into a tea shop and ask for a cream cake. I am thinking of a vanilla slice but the waitress brings me a chocolate eclair. I am disappointed. However if she had asked what type of cream cake I wanted she could either have brought me what I wanted, or constituted a new reality for me by explaining that as well as vanilla slices she had chocolate eclairs. Whilst this is a trivial example, it illustrates an idea which has been used in nursing to explore patients' experience of a range of phenomena including labour pain (Kelpin, 1992), courage in the face of chronic illness (Haase, 1987), death (Gullickson, 1993), caring (Forrest, 1989), and breathing for sufferers of asthma (Clarke, 1992). By discovering the meaning of these phenomena for a series of individuals, a new understanding of the experience can be constituted by nurses, and thus facilitate assessment and care of future patients experiencing the same phenomenon, but all the time recognizing that each individual will experience unique nuances.

Rosemarie Parse (1981, 1987, 1992b, 1994, 1995) has

made a major contribution to the naturalistic exploration of human experience in nursing, by using phenomenological philosophy in the construction of her Theory of Human Becoming. In this theory she introduces the concept of co-creation of reality. By this she means that human beings are in continuous interaction with the whole universe, including the people within it, and construct their reality from the choices made available to them. In relation to nursing, one of the roles of the nurse is to help the patient disclose, to themselves and the nurse, their current reality, that is the objects of their thoughts. The nurse then introduces to the patient a new set of ideas. Both the nurse and patient can then construct a new reality using ideas from both their original realities.

Santopinto (1989) describes this process in the care of young women whose 'relentless drive to be ever thinner' is labelled anorexia nervosa. The aim was first to uncover the experience of the phenomenon for the patient. The nurse then suggested to the patient new ways of looking at the phenomenon, and finally, practice propositions which presented a new reality were identified. For example, one of the experiences that the patient had was that she did not know who she was as her perceptions differed from what her friends told her. She felt socially incompetent whereas her friends told her she was out-going and fun to be with. The nurse suggested that the conflict opened up the opportunity for the patient to find out who she really was by using both her own perceptions and those of her friends to form a new picture of herself, rather than struggle to decide which of the conflicting ideas was true. The practice proposition was that 'struggling to be who you want to be means finding new ways of picturing yourself together with your friends'.

From her *Theory of Human Becoming*, Parse (1995) has also developed a research methodology for nursing which relies on phenomenological philosophy as its basis. By doing this she has demonstrated that academic rigour can be used in conducting first-order research to explore and describe phenomena as they are experienced by individuals. In the quest for knowledge nursing has relied heavily on science, albeit in both paradigms. However, there are other types of knowledge which, if one lays aside the assumptions of science, can add to the understanding of nursing and nursing practice. An examination of the relationship between theory and knowledge in nursing will help to demonstrate this.

Torres (1990) suggests that theory construction is an intellectual process by which relationships between phenomena are sought through comparison and experimentation, and Craig (1980) describes it as a scientific process. Chinn and Jacobs (1987) define theory as a set of concepts, definitions, and propositions that project a systematic view of phenomena by designing specific interrelationships among concepts for the purpose of describing, explaining and predicting. In relation to nursing (Smith, 1981) suggests that nursing science is a unique mix of other sciences with the uniqueness lying in the mix. Adam (1987) however holds the view that theory in any discipline is developed by asking questions that differ substantially from those asked in other disciplines. She argues that nursing has become interested in theory development not only to acquire knowledge for practice, and contribute to the knowledge base relating to health matters, but because of a desire to be recognized as a legitimate member of the scientific community. Powers and Knapp (1990) emphasize that theory is tentative; it is not reality but a model of reality based on assumptions about the phenomena being explained. One of the problems of theory in practice however is that it is used as if it were reality, therefore excluding the nuances of human uniqueness. For example theories of human response to loss have been developed which, if used too rigidly to inform practice, may exclude the possibility that some people are glad of the death of a loved one and thus grieve differently (Smith, 1994).

Silva (1977) agrees that the aim of theory is to describe, understand, predict, control and explain, and that theory is a set of related statements derived from scientific data, from which hypotheses emerge to be tested. The process of generating theory, she suggests is research, which may be conducted using methodologies from any of the scientific paradigms. Theory is also tested through research methodology and it is only after rigorous testing that theory can be said to become new knowledge within the discipline concerned. Even then, however, it is recognized that research can at best only lead to a high degree of probability and never to absolute proof (Chalmers, 1982). The philosophy of art however suggests that art is the expression of certain values, such as caring, compassion, humour and honesty, with an expectation that an emotional response will be elicited. If nursing is created with a recognition of human uniqueness, then the expectation will be that the responses to nursing will be unique to the individual experiencing it, rather than predictable.

In terms of the relationship between nursing art and science Peplau (1988) declares that both are essential, and that the values of each can inform and nourish the other. She describes how these values compare, for example art values subjectivity and involvement, whereas science values objectivity and detachment. She states that art is always an expressive response, and emphasizes this as a process in nursing. She acknowledges that whilst nursing is not a scientific endeavour but a practice, the components of science can be found within it, for example in data collection, planning and evaluation of care. The problem with this type of explanation is that art and science are viewed as different entities making up nursing.

Imagine, for one moment a landscape artist out on the hills. Her tools are the paint brushes and canvass, the elements she weaves into the painting are colour and perspective. She always paints landscapes, but no two are alike. Likewise the nurse using scientific knowledge and technological hardware as tools, mixes the elements of nursing, manual dexterity, interpersonal skills, and so on, to create nursing. She always creates nursing but it is always unique. In the same way that each painting created by the landscape artist is more than the sum of the paints, the artist's knowledge of the physics of colour and perspective, and the artist's intuition, so nursing is a distinct entity which is different from, and greater than, the sum of science and technology, and the nurses tacit knowledge, within it. Thus to know nursing involves more than an understanding of the 'ologies', sociology, physiology, biology and so on. It also involves more than the application of these to practice.

Carper (1978) outlined four patterns of knowing important to nursing theory. She acknowledged empirics, or scientific knowledge and she argued that the highly integrated abstract and systematic explanations of scientific enquiry remain an ideal towards which nursing strives. Personal knowledge (sometimes termed tacit knowledge) Carper describes as the most problematic, being difficult to master and teach, but possibly the most essential. She describes it as a knowledge of self, and suggests that a nurse cannot acknowledge and respect the uniqueness of each individual unless she knows her own uniqueness. If the nurse has this knowledge then interactions with patients will become authentic and reciprocal rather than the nurse being in authority. Carper says that this kind of knowledge cannot be described or even experienced, it can only be actualized.

Ethics, the knowledge of morality, is a pattern of knowing, necessary if nurses are to make decisions about how to act with each patient and in each circumstance. Aesthetics, or the art of nursing is a pattern of knowing in which the type of knowledge is expressive and made visible through action, rather than published in a written form. However, for this reason, it is only the patient involved in the action, or interaction, who witnesses the aesthetic knowledge. The requirement that art has an audience was discussed in relation to what constitutes art and Carper's view of aesthetic knowledge suggests that it is indeed the patient who is the audience for nursing art, and as Lumby (1991) suggests that nurses, as true artists, are not only willing, but see it as essential, to share their artistic performance with others.

Smith, M. (1992) acknowledges Carper's statement that her patterns of knowing are all necessary, interrelated, interdependent and overlapping, but suggests that it is only if this is ignored that knowledge can be categorized as Carper does. Smith argues that knowing is a holistic and integrative process, and that whilst it may come from a variety of sources such as science, arts, humanities, life experiences, perceptions and reflections, the threads are selected by the individual and reflect their personal beliefs and values. Even in science she argues the researcher selects the subject area, methodology, and method of presentation which reflects their personal preferences. Thus she suggests that personal knowing is not one of four patterns of knowing but has a central and primary place in all knowing. This implies that nursing practice is the expression of personal knowing. Benner (1984) supports this by suggesting that theory derived in the scientific paradigms acts as a guide which can enable nurses to ask the right questions and she gives examples such as the grieving process, and mother–infant bonding to illustrate this. However, she goes on to say that any nurse experienced in working with these theories finds differences, or nuances, that the formal theory fails to express. Thus, the expert nurse goes on to use intuition, or personal knowing, to fill the gaps.

Benner and Tanner (1987) suggest that it is intuition (discussed in full in Chapter 5), which they define as understanding without a rationale, that is the process by which the most experienced nurses, whom they define as expert, make the decisions which inform their practice. They suggest that intuition has traditionally been viewed not as knowledge but as the basis of irrational acts, guesswork and even supernatural influences. However they argue that it is intuition that distinguishes human thinking from that of a machine. They argue that intuition should not be dismissed simply because there appears to be a lack of concrete evidence supporting a decision to take a particular course of action. Indeed they go on to point out that sometimes measured scientific data does not give the full picture to support action but that a subsequent failure, therefore, to act on 'intuition' because of its uncertainty, could have serious consequences. This has long been recognized by our medical colleagues who use the term 'clinical judgement' to justify actions or opinions for which they cannot articulate a scientific base. Yet according to Benner and Tanner (1987) these medical colleagues, as well as expert nurses themselves, are the very people who devalue intuition in nursing practice.

Clarke (1986) suggests that intuitive knowledge can only be obtained through reflection on the performance of the action every time it is carried out, in order to build up knowledge of the range of possible responses. She argues that nursing activity is primary, and that theory arises from it and modifies it. Nursing theory thus derives from reflection on practice and the questions arising from that reflection. Dickoff and James (1968) express this by suggesting that, as nursing is a profession, and that as a professional is a doer who shapes reality, then the appropriate theory for nursing is what they describe as situation-producing theory, that is theory which is action-oriented. The link here can be made with the nurse as co-creator of reality with the patient. As creativity is one of the features of art this again suggests that the nurse as artist may use science and technology as tools but that nursing as a creative activity is art, and that which is created is a work of art.

Benner (1984) suggests that, after much reflection (a concept addressed in full in Chapter 6) the expert nurse, with an enormous background of experience, now has an intuitive grasp of each situation. In this way reflection can provide the nurse with the knowledge to act on intuition without necessarily being able to articulate that this is what is taking place. Thus the scientific knowledge base is left unarticulated whilst the art is created intuitively.

English (1993) however criticizes the work of Benner. He explains that the only way Benner obtained a sample of 'expert' nurses, whose characteristics she then described, was by peer assessment, i.e. those whom peers said were expert. English suggests that more formal criteria should have been applied. He also commented on her suggestion that expert nurses cannot articulate their knowledge. English feels that this means only expert nurses will understand other expert nurses so they become almost like a 'secret society' whose 'rites of passage' are not available to outsiders. This also links with the problem he identifies as Benner's failure to make explicit the actual catalyst which stimulates the move from the proficient nurse to the expert nurse on the continuum of skills acquisition, and the problem of why some people following the model will never, according to Benner, become experts. He also comments on Benner's failure to provide negative cases in her descriptions of intuition, and examine possible examples of the process in nurses who have not achieved the status of 'expert'. A problem with the work of English is that he makes no reference to the role of reflection in Benner's model and it only becomes clear in his conclusion that he bases his work on the assumption that nursing should be founded on scientific knowledge and empirical research if it is to become a research-based profession and that the 'hunches' of Benner's experts are not acceptable. Thus he appears to omit artistry as a feature of professional practice. Picture again our landscape artist mixing colours on the palate. This artist does not measure out the exact amount from each tube of paint to obtain the desired colour mix. From experience the painter intuitively squeezes the tubes of paint, mixes the colour and adds a little of this, and a little of that, until the exact nuance of colour is achieved for purpose. Each mix will be unique to the needs of painting being undertaken. Likewise, the nurse can intuitively use a unique mix of nursing skills to create the nuance of nursing required for the patient in her care.

Rew and Barrow (1987) suggest that, far from being inappropriate as an aspect of nursing knowledge, intuition is recognized as a component of the perceived view of science, and is of importance in enabling nurses to respond to new situations creatively, using imagination and abstract thinking. In a study of 85 years of nursing literature, Rew and Barrow (1987) found that intuition, or related terms such as empathy, nursing art, and instinct, sustained over time the characteristics of being related to the intangibles in nurse–patient relationships, and to holism. However the link between intuition and nursing artistry died out after the first 30 years, only to reappear 20 years later. Their findings suggest that whilst nursing has traditionally valued artistry, this was, for a time at least, displaced by the quest for objective knowledge.

The risk, if artistry is neglected in professional practice, is that practitioners will focus so much on rules that their patients may become dehumanized cases. Jarvis (1992) explains that because all actions are performed within a context there is always an element of probability in terms of the outcomes. Thus the value of the theory brought to that context from the classroom will depend on how able the practitioner is to use it within the action. If patients are dehumanized and theory is not related to the context, then actions become, according to Jarvis a mindless repetition which becomes self-destructive. It will be practitioners functioning in this way who, whilst they may have extensive knowledge, will never become Benner's experts. Thus action will remain creative only as long as the unique individuality of each patient is central to the context of that action.

Holmes (1991) argues that whilst a great deal of attention has been paid to the philosophy of science and theory generated through scientific research, the theory of art and aesthetics is not well developed. He suggests that part of the problem lies in the fact that aesthetic knowledge cannot be articulated and therefore is not always acknowledged as 'real' knowledge. Where artistry in nursing is discussed it is often viewed as the process which leads to scientifically measurable outcomes. Lumby (1991) states that nurses deny their art; whilst the evidence presented in this chapter suggests that this is not entirely true, there is no doubt that there is a lack of clarity regarding the nature of nursing as an art. Whilst attempts are made to measure the value of nursing in quantifiable terms, its true value, as an art form, must remain private and unmeasured, because it is viewed by each individual patient as if having a private audience.

It is in keeping with modern art theory to consider nursing as an art form. Stecker (1993) outlined two recent attempts to define art which can be used to support the view that nursing is art. The first, known as the *open-concept theory*, suggests that an item of art cannot be defined as such in isolation, because art is an open-concept to which specific conditions or criteria cannot be applied. Classification of one item or activity as art must be made by its resemblance to other items or activities that have been similarly classified. Thus to examine nursing in the light of characteristics present in say, painting or dance, is a legitimate way of deciding whether nursing too is art. Critics of this theory of course, ask what properties are acceptable in this comparison, and how great the differences must be to suggest the new item or activity is not art. However the comparisons I have made between nursing and other art forms, throughout this chapter, may be accepted by supporters of this theory, as evidence enough that nursing is art.

Secondly, the *institutional theory* of art suggests that art is defined by its acceptance as art within a particular culture or society, and that therefore art is a sociological fact, rather than a cross-cultural reality. Using this theory it is less easy to justify that nursing is art. There are many nurses, some of whose views I have represented within this chapter, who do identify nursing as art. However, nursing is not yet accepted as art by the 'artworld', by that I mean art historians, academics and teachers as well as practitioners of various art forms. We do not see articles about nursing in art journals, or in the textbooks of students of art. Nor do we see nursing situated within the humanities departments of universities. However, this theory suggests that it is possible for nursing to become recognized as an art form within our, or perhaps another, time or culture.

In summary then, if nursing is accepted as an art form, then science is part of its knowledge base, along with the nurses tacit knowledge, and technology the tools of the trade for the nurse, just as a knowledge of colour and perspective, and a box of paints and brushes, are the knowledge and tools of the painter. Then just as the picture created by the painter hangs on the gallery wall for the public to view, so nursing is displayed in the wards, clinics and homes of the sick, for patients to perceive. It is not, in the art gallery, the artists knowledge, or tools that are important, but the painting which is created, that is the work of art. In the same way it is not nursing theory, science or technology that is nursing. Nursing is the thing which the nurse creates using this knowledge and these tools. It is unique to each nurse artist creating it, and unique to each member of its audience.

CHAPTER 3   *You seem to be suggesting that science and technology matter, and that nursing cannot do without them.*

CHAPTER 2   *That's right, but there is more to it than that, isn't there?*

CHAPTER 3   *The 'more to it' is the caring. I think we need to deconstruct the cold, marble pedestal, on which science and technology have stood for so long. We must co-create, with caring, something new, so that the beauty of the marble is not lost, but it is no longer cold and impersonal.*

CHAPTER 2   *In other words, we are* reconstructing *nursing, and presenting a new face of the cube.*

CHAPTER 3   *What you did was turn the cube to give us a glimpse of this new face; I want to get to the heart and soul of it, and its place in healing. . . .*

ARTISTRY OF CARING: HEART AND SOUL OF NURSING

Jean Watson

It's the art that sustains me in a profession that many of my colleagues contemplate leaving. It's the art that expresses what drew me to nursing in the first place and connects me with every other nurse. I submit that the heart of nursing is the art of nursing, and to quote Wordsworth, 'we' have to give our hearts away . . .

(Veneta Masson, 1987)

A focus on the artistry of caring summons forth the heart and soul of nursing. It seems that during this century, the caring, healing arts of nursing have been somewhat in retreat. We seem to have pushed away these caring-making arts to yield to the harsh acts pressed into our busy institutional lives. Perhaps the fact that the artistry of caring, and even nursing arts, have been in retreat during this century, does not deny the fact that they are now needed again to metamorphose back into our soulless systems.

This chapter will examine two themes: The age of post-modernism and its influence on how nursing understands its own knowledge base; and the art and artistry of caring as the heart and soul of nursing.

♦

THE AGE OF POST-MODERNISM

The phrase 'post-modernism' is a bit ambiguous and hard to define, although almost every field of human activity seems to be engaged in issues related to post-modernist thought (Watson, 1995). Toulmin (1990) suggests that post-modern thought is defined by both the beginning and end of Modernity. Tarnas (1993), however, suggests that post-modernism marks the end of the western world view and its dominant idea of one reality, and the replacement with a world view of multiple realities. Lather (1991) offers a feminist definition of post-modernism as

> .... a response across disciplines to the contemporary crisis of profound uncertainty brought about by the crash of modern hope of rationality and technology to solve human dilemmas....
>
> (Lather, 1991, p. 20)

I have proposed (Watson, 1995) that the western world view of modernism, which contrasts with post-modernism, has come to suggest that human reasoning is value-neutral, and is concerned with control and dominance of one world view for predicting reality and sustaining our notions of reality. Knowledge within this modern, western world view is equated with science, and science in turn is equated with reality. Within the understanding of what reality is, the western world view of modernism has come to place its value in facts over meaning; in scientific evidence over the spiritual or intuitive and in the physical over non-physical or metaphysical.

All aspects of human endeavour, whether it be art, literature, music, quantum physics, philosophy and even nursing are involved in a shift away from modernism to post-modernism. In nursing, this paradigm shift can be seen in Fawcett (1993a) who described an organismic and mechanistic world view, and in Parse (1981, 1992b) who suggests simultaneity and totality paradigms which change our approaches toward human beings and health.

What is clear is that there is a growing mistrust or lack of confidence in traditional Western dualist conceptual systems. Lather (1991) suggests that the ideas underpinning dualism

> ...which continues to dominate Western thought are inadequate for understanding a world of multiple causes and effects interacting in complex and non-linear ways....
>
> (Lather, 1991, p. 21)

It is the challenge to this notion of dualism that has enabled post-modernism to shift our understanding of who we are and what is possible.

The rise in post-modernism has been most evident in Europe and is represented in philosophy, in the attempt by phenomenology to understand the human experience, in the advent of critical and interpretive hermeneutics, the rise of feminism and on to the development of deconstructionism and reconstructionism (Watson, 1995).

The end result of these new ways of viewing the world is that rationality has ceased to be at the centre of our understanding of reality, a dramatic shift in our understanding of what is to count as knowledge and an uprising against 'all the "experts" who . . . speak for or on behalf of others.' (Lather, 1991, p. 23).

Uris (1993) suggests that this post-modernist challenge of knowledge and expertise questions the notion of a single correct approach to knowledge development or a single idea of truth or meaning of reality. The idea of one true story about reality is rejected. This ontological and epistemological shift focuses not on knowledge for its own sake, but rather, emphasizes context, connection, relationships, multiplicity, openness, paradox, process and the mysteries of the human experience of 'being-in-the world' (Watson, 1995).

Toulmin (1990) quoted Yeats (1865–1939), and described his phrase 'things fall apart; the centre cannot hold', as a phrase which describes the essences of post-modernism. This notion of 'falling apart' I previously described as the downside of post-modernism; commonly referred to as *deconstruction*. Deconstruction is about old ideas of knowledge and action 'falling apart'. This deconstruction emerged from the human despair brought about by society's dependence on modern scientific and technological advances, the knowledge explosion and quests for new meaning of the human condition (Watson, 1995).

Post-modern thought has now generated new questions about humanity, nature and survival. Through deconstruction, 'things fall apart and the centre can no longer hold'. This acknowledges that there is no one way of knowing or being or experiencing reality. The rationalist model ceases to explain; we move away from problems which can be fixed, towards multiple solutions with endless possibilities for what might be.

Deconstruction may be liberating and give birth to new

notions of reality, but socially, it also leads to human and environmental confusion and even moral void, and these, indeed, have been features of post-modern society, yet post-modernism had also led to a new quest for meaning in the cosmos (Tarnas, 1993). In nursing, it has led to a new and transformative paradigm of caring in the human health experience (Newman, 1992). This new paradigm of caring which emerged out of post-modern thought identified a moral foundation for nursing and an imperative of human caring with respect to the human health experience. The post-modern evolution out of modernism has led to a shift away from what Fawcett (1993b) called 'reaction world view' into a 'reciprocal world view'.

♦

FROM DECON-STRUCTION TO CON-STRUCTION

From the darkness of deconstruction has emerged a new light of reconstruction, the positive side of post-modernism. In moving from Fawcett's Reaction Worldview towards a Reciprocal Worldview and perhaps into a Simultaneous Worldview, we also move away from the dualist idea of knowledge and experience and the domination of rationality, technological controls and notions of knowledge based on science which the age of modernity thrust upon us. The reconstruction of reality which is emerging has acknowledged new notions of reality, had led to a search for meaning which invites personal experiences as its own truth and has allowed for the concept of connectedness to shape human relationships. This is an historic point in the evolution of humanity in general, and in nursing specifically. It is calling for a radical re-thinking of constructing and reconstructing ourselves and our worlds. The centre cannot hold in the chaos of deconstruction and reconstruction, but we can re-create, or co-create, a new centre, a new form of knowledge and human experience which will ultimately lead us towards a higher evolution. This is especially true with respect to nursing, its caring–healing process, its diverse ways of knowing.

So what are the post-modern implications for nursing knowledge? The age of modernity and rationality excluded certain ideas of knowledge because that knowledge did not fit into the thinking of Modernity, science and technology. Post-modernism in nursing is heralded by the fact that certain knowledge which was previously excluded has now been reconsidered in order that we can reconnect with the human condition (Smith, M., 1992). Some of this knowledge goes beyond the physical, material, and factual of the Modern era. Some of this new idea of knowledge is a re-awakening of the moral consciousness in nursing, of compassion that moves like a chain of concentric circles (Noddings, 1984) from self-care, to caring for others, to caring for the environment, to nature, to caring for and being part of an ever-evolving universe which we are co-creating.

Even though this new era of post-modern thought has yet to be fully defined/re-defined, nursing needs to yield, and indeed is yielding, to post-modernism. Contemporary nursing theories are demonstrating evidence of post-modern directions in understanding nursing knowledge (Rogers, 1989; Newman, 1992; Newman et al, 1991; Parse, 1992b; Sarter, 1988; Watson, 1984, 1988) even though these are not overtly labelled as post-modern. Shared themes are emerging (Sarter, 1988) which are redefining nursing knowledge and demonstrating a shift from modern to post-modern. As nursing finds its place in this emerging post-modern world, with its downside of deconstruction and its positive side of reconstruction, nursing is learning to live with open-endedness, ambiguity, dynamic construction incessantly questioned, endlessly self-revising, a floating and moving river of its own life.

Part of the reconstruction which is emerging is an uncovering and reconstruction of nursing's most ancient caring–healing–health knowledge and practice, the artistry of caring.

♦

THE HEART AND SOUL OF NURSING

Modern medical care systems have created war-like metaphors to deal with human health–illness experiences in order to battle, conquer, conquest and cure at all costs, usually through detached technological approaches – approaches that stand alone and apart from any attention to the human life and the life spirit.

With respect to the artistry of caring, do we stop to consider that nursing arts manifest through connecting with the poetry of human existence, through myth, life story, through all ways of being human? It is the arts and the artistry of connecting with life spirit, the life force, of self and other within the greater universe that art offers a ready contrast to the mundane of daily living, of mechanical institutional practices. As Masson (1987, p. 187) called out to us:

> To nurse – really, truly – is art, and our art holds the power we need to unite us, keep us going, move us forward. It's time, high time, to unleash it.

In spite of the decline of nursing arts during this century, the caring–healing art of nursing is emerging within a new framework for healing practices. We might ask if in all the dark institutions designed for sick care, could there be a more critical contribution to the human soul than the caring art/act in nursing? The public itself is now questing for wholeness, care of the soul.

The caring art re-emergence in nursing at the turn of this century is an affirmation of rebirth, a request for healing; perhaps a counterpoint to isolation, detached treatments, and sterile technology. Caring arts and science are helping to restore an ecological balance between art and science, between human and nature – helping to make right what is currently in disorder.

The artistry of caring draws from the same source as life itself; from human encounter, engaging with the indelible stories of people, of caring moments of connecting through eyes, touch, sound, space, spirit itself. Such engaging moments of caring touch the human soul and provide a reflection into human existence – the personal and the profound, serving as mirror and image into humanity. A caring moment is art serving all at once, connecting an individual spirit with the universal – art serving as mediator between matter and spirit, between suffering and compassion.

Thus, the caring–healing arts and aesthetics of nursing's practices differ from the exclusive medical cures in ways we cannot imagine. Caring and the arts touch the human soul, which calls forth the continually mysterious emergence of beauty and spirit from matter. Art cannot be extinguished in the human mind and soul.

In considering and re-considering art and aesthetics of nursing we take back what has been increasingly disowned during the 20th century and during this so-called 'modern' era. The lures throughout the rise of Modernity and the peak of western science in medicine and nursing have resulted in a neglect of our own practices and the nature of our very arts in caring.

We affirm nursing arts as one of the oldest arts of caring – caring for the infirm, the wounded, those most vulnerable and suffering from mind–body–spirit severing; those most in need of healing approaches of the arts. It is human art which seeks to restore wholeness associated with the imbalance created by the concrete and existential pain of human experiences of health and illness.

The art of caring evokes the most human and humane processes of sustaining and expanding our being. It creates opportunities for full expression of self as the ultimate caring art/act. Caring is relational and a caring moment transcends and transforms both the one caring and the one cared for (Watson, 1988); not unlike a work of art both transcending and transforming the viewer. Any nurse who has stood in that sacred place where they have truly, artistically touched the life spirit, the life force of another, understands the power and beauty, the aesthetic arrest of the connection – soul to soul.

The artistry of caring is soulful; the artistry of caring is soul to soul connecting; the artistry of caring is soul care. It is more homoeopathic in its workings – often acting as a natural pharmaceutical, rather than an allopathic (Moore, 1992). The caring arts of nursing sense that for every physical ailment there is a metaphysical, soul-felt, mirror. The human caring process recognizes that artful acts of expression tap into archetypes, myths, rituals, poetry, music, movement, meanings – symbolic and real–that cleanse the mind and soul, potentiate wholeness and healing patterns and process that have their own natural will and direction.

The most powerful aspect of art of caring in nursing is that it involves care of the soul. The work of Thomas Moore (1992) by that title reminds us of the fact that care of the soul never ends, it is not a short-term problem to be fixed and solved and not to be dealt with again. Rather the art of soul-care takes the form of a circle, reflecting and re-learning, re-working, re-creating meaning out of the raw material of living, exploring it, turning the experience over and over, telling ourselves the story again and again, each time with depth of meaning and insight to see the themes, the myths, the meanings that we create and which circle in our lives.

One who cares for the soul, which is what I submit nursing and the artistry of caring–healing attend to, often are helping self and other to recover, remember parts that have been lost, dealing with aspects we are protecting ourselves against, viewing and embracing the shadow we reject, in order to more clearly see the light.

Art of nursing becomes a means for considering the soul, the life spirit of the one, without judging, appreciating and accepting the eccentricities and unexpected tendencies of the soul. Care of the soul and arts/aesthetics may evoke the not-so-normal, the unusual expression of life. As Moore (1992) puts is, sometimes deviation from the usual is a special revelation of truth. A facade of normality can be hiding the soullessness of the standardizing of experience and of institutions, be they educational or clinical settings.

Our work in nursing would change radically if we thought about, developed, and re-owned the art/aesthetics of nursing and seriously regarded it as an on-going caring process, rather than continuing to hitch our energy and our development to the scientific quest for cure of the body physical, at all costs to the soul and to the arts.

Were we to consider again the human art and artistry of caring in our practices of nursing, we might then take time to watch, to listen, to create sacred space for birthing of healing and wholeness as the passage and process of the caring art/act unravels and reveals the deeper mysteries lying within daily turmoils of disease, pathology, pain and suffering (Moore, 1992). Care of the soul as the art/act of caring involves paradox and subjective revelations of the essence and spirit of each person, thereby recovering a sense of sacredness of each life and each caring moment, not just sacredness, but the recovering of a sense of the unfathomable mystery in the heart of each life (Moore, 1992).

Until and unless nursing focuses–refocuses nursing on its ancient and contemporary caring–healing arts, away from its exclusive 20th century Modern science model of standardizing nursing process and procedures and medical treatment and institutional/bureaucratic regimes, the mystery will continue to shrink, the human soul will continue to be decentered and our institutional darkness will continue to remain soulless; nursing itself will continue to unwittingly perpetuate acts and practices where there can be no light for wholeness and healing, rather there may be acts of cruelty; more pain, more suffering (Chinn and Watson, 1994).

Nursing in the 20th century separated art from science and both were separated from spirituality. Projecting itself into the 21st century, nursing is called upon to radically re-imagine itself if it is to restore the artistry and science of its practices that are converging to re-integrate mind, body, spirit and to go beyond art and science. In this revision, the art and artistry of our human acts as shared acts, as complete art/acts, that unite rather than divide, must be seen again as one. This new paradigm of art and human science brings us to the end of modern, material nursing as we have known it. New visions, new vocabulary, and new traditions are being developed that reach back into the finest of Nightingale's (1859) art of nursing, and leap forward towards greater possibilities of what might be (Chinn and Watson, 1994).

So, as nursing transforms itself for the next millennium we can let go of lots of things that no longer work, but we must remember, that if we give away, and turn away, from the art of caring, from the artistry of being human, we give away the heart and soul of nursing. We give away what it means to sustain human caring and healing for life itself. The reverse is in the deep discovery: ultimately, it is through the artistry of human caring that we heal the heart and soul of humanity across time.

In summary then, the age of modernism gave us a belief that science, technology and rationality would solve human dilemmas. The realization that rationality and technology does not have the ability to provide all answers lead to the era of uncertainty and a new quest for understanding about truth and reality. Post-modernism is a response from all walks of life and all disciplines, including nursing, to find new explanations and meanings. Reality and truth are no longer objectively defined. Caring and healing, connecting with each other and with the universe and creating wholeness is a part of the new reality and new truth.

Conversation

CHAPTER 4   *What you have said is stunning. Through the beauty of the language you used, I saw before me a vivid expression of nursing.*

CHAPTER 3   *I'm glad, because I intended just that; to express what art and artistry in nursing might be. Using the language of post-modernism may be new to some nurses, but it can also give them a vision of how nursing can be.*

CHAPTER 4   *Yes, you've created a splendid backdrop for my presentation of the values within nursing.*

CHAPTER 3   *Thank you. The artistry of caring has so many facets to it: heart; soul; feelings; healing; connecting; as well as values.*

CHAPTER 4   *That sounds right to me, but it is also about opposites, contradictions, and wholeness, and how these might be looked at in new ways....*

NURSING AS A MORAL ART

Verena Tschudin

Look with thine ears

(King Lear, Act 4, Scene 6.1)

To hear with eyes belongs to love's fine wit

(Sonnet XXIII)

There is a certain inconsistency in the title of this chapter. Can *nursing* be moral and artistic? Is it not the *individuals* who are moral (or not) and who practise the art (when they are moral) of nursing?

Contradictions, opposites, symbols, meanings and interpretations all play very important parts in nursing, as in all spheres of life. I have often been challenged by such concepts, both personally and professionally. Because I believe that this is more than just an individual quirk, I will present a few of these concepts in this chapter with the aim of considering art, morality and nursing from various angles for enlightenment, perhaps enjoyment, possibly for orientation, but not as a means to finding solutions, simply presenting, as it were, the faces of a cube.

By their very nature, contradictions, symbols and opposites are often hidden or unconscious factors, with unexpected and untamed powers. They reveal themselves differently in different circumstances and in different places and cultures. This may mean that they are only partly understood. This could be a justification for any ignorance or one-sided interpretation on my part; it could also be due to their tricksterish nature, for what to me may be profound or exciting may to you be opaque, meaningless or missing the point.

♦

ARCHETYPES

The psychologist C.G. Jung (1875–1961) is perhaps best known for two aspects of his work, namely the descriptions of the 'shadow' (1946) and the 'archetypes' (1964). Shadow and archetype are sometimes used in association with each other, sometimes separately.

According to Stewart (1992, p. 252), the 'shadow involves the personal unconscious, instincts, the collective unconscious, and archetypes' which are made evident in 'both negative and positive projections, which are powerful and potentially destructive', but which a person can be helped to own, accept and integrate, and therefore also analyse in order to break their compulsive hold.

Jung (1964, p. 57) described archetypes as 'archaic remnants', 'primordial images', 'collective images' (p.69), or 'collective representations' (p.42). Archetypes express themselves in dreams and particularly in mythology, giving the possibility to see analogies and to use and understand symbols. Here they can represent the shadow and make it accessible. For instance, a pregnant woman dreamed of two trees growing in her garden and found later that day, that she was expecting twins.

The terms 'shadow' and 'archetype' have strong negative or obscure connotations in popular understanding. This is largely due to the fear of their powers. When both shadow and archetype are more understood, they become positive powers also. I will concentrate here on two archetypes: that of the nurse, and of Cassandra.

The nurse

In symbolic language – in dreams, tales, stories, and the personal unconscious – the nurse represents both the woman and the mother who nourishes. (As this is in symbolic language, gender is not as differentiated as it is in practice.) There can sometimes be a confusion between a child's (wet) nurse and a sick nurse, but essentially the nurse is identified with the 'anima', that is, with the unconscious female figure in a man's psyche. There the anima connotes mother, sister, wife, daughter, the 'wise' woman, witch, the 'angel in white' and female ancestry and progeny generally. The nurse nourishes, protects and strengthens both physical growth (the wet nurse) and promotes emotional growth (the sick nurse). The nurse is thus a healer in the broadest sense of the word, restoring, binding wounds, soothing heated brows, and 'making good'. 'In myth the nurse may be symbolic of Nature herself looking after the abandoned hero' (Chetwynd, 1982, p. 291).

But the archetype itself has its shadow, and in this the nurse is the woman who withholds healing, restoration, nourishment and growth, destroys rather than builds, and denies autonomy by keeping patients in a 'baby' condition. This is often evident in the names patients are given: 'pet', 'lovey', etc. This is the shadow which women, who are nurses, may unconsciously use with sinister effect. This may come as a surprise to many nurses. But, Bradshaw (1994) cites a patient who after a stroke, was 'on several occasions left in a cold bath and forgotten on the commode for more than half an hour. He was left by a porter in a wheelchair outside the X-ray department, when a nursing sister appeared and, without acknowledging him, shouted over his head "Who has left this man here?" Two nurses made his bed around him without interrupting their conversation'.

That nurses have on occasion been cruel to be kind is quite acceptable, but deliberately withholding healing and nourishment to those in their care, and even smothering their attempts at autonomy, seems preposterous. Yet the principle of the archetype is not unlike much else in nature, that is, it has to have an opposite in order to function. Electricity only works because it has a negative and a positive charge; a day consists of a period of night and a period of day. In the same way, psychology recognizes the positive and the negative aspects of being; they complement each other. Thus the shadow of the nurse is as necessary as its radiant opposite.

It is possible to look back over the history of nursing and see moments when the shadow of withholding care (not the carelessness just mentioned) has been powerfully at work. Florence Nightingale had spent most of her life fighting good causes, speaking and writing on behalf of patients and nurses. But she totally opposed the state registration of nurses. At a crucial moment of development, this woman of influence withheld her support. At various stages nurses have taken industrial action, often against advice, and usually being castigated for doing so. But did they need to withhold their services in order to gain something? Does the need of the few have to yield to the need of the many?

Many nurses know to their cost that when they feel compelled to speak up about some practice which they judge to be contrary to their conscience, their colleagues' support vanishes like ice in the heat. This text is being written at a time when nurses in Britain are fighting to be given the same pay rises as other health care workers, that is, over six percent, but have only been promised two percent by the government. This has united nurses to fight their corner. It remains to be seen if in a decade or so this will have been a wise move. It may have been; on the other hand, it may also have been a move away from conscious political action and local and community involvement. Here, too, nurses may be withholding their strengths.

Some of these shadowy actions may have been conscious decisions, but it is also possible that they are unconscious and symbolic actions, geared to defending a known stance. Nurses have great power: there are many of them in the country; they are associated with healing and comforting; their symbolic image is strong as the women who are 'there' when needed. When those palpable and symbolic presences are withdrawn, nurses can create terror and sickness.

Individual nurses reflect and represent what nursing does as a profession. One of the essential insights from psychology which most of us have to learn at some stage is that whatever we would do or be to others, we have to do or be to ourselves first. This is particularly true of the professions with strong symbolic images: doctors have to learn to doctor themselves ('Physician, heal thyself'); priests have to learn to be priests to themselves; judges have to be judges to themselves first before they can be judges of others. In just the same way, nurses have to learn to nurse themselves before they can truly nurse other people. This is not something which is learned in basic nursing education. It may not be until many years into nursing that individual nurses come to this insight.

The most common answer to the question why someone wants to be a nurse is, 'to help other people'. Is the real motive (coming from the shadow) for this desire to help, a psychological need to be helped oneself? What went on in the early life of a child that when it grows up it is left with remnants of memories of being hurt, wounded, left un-cared? These wounds cry for help, and clearly, the mothers and nannies who should have supplied the need, cannot do so now if they could not do it earlier. The search for the restorer, healer, comforter, nourisher, is so strong that it translates into action to the extent of dedicating one's life to nursing and healing. We try to find the meaning of our lives through what we do, and it may be that when one day we realize that we have been seeking job satisfaction, we have in fact been seeking psychological satisfaction. Then perhaps we do not need to carry on being nurses; but we would then be much more effective nurses. We could give and not be concerned about what we get at the level of the ego.

The archetypal shadow may have been responsible for our not getting what we needed as a child, but the archetypal nurse of the psyche made sure that through actual nursing we became a more whole – *holistic* – person. Learning to be a nurse to oneself may be painful; it may also, for those who are nurses, bring the most liberating insight. This insight does not come on request, but unbidden and as a surprise. When it does come, it is, however, usually most welcome.

What happens at the level of the personal must, I believe, also happen collectively and professionally. But it is not often at the moment of crisis or need that an insight appears. It is in retrospect, perhaps with a throw-away remark, that a leap forward in the history of nursing is made. This seems to be happening now with Nightingale's famous remark that 'hospitals should do the sick no harm'. Suddenly this phrase has taken on the status of the war-cry for nurses who are concerned about what happens, humanly speaking, to patients. This could only happen because the ground had been prepared enough and the collective psyche and unconscious was ready for this insight. The ground is made ready by reflection and awareness at many levels: that is where nursing becomes moral, and an art.

Cassandra In 1852 Florence Nightingale wrote an essay entitled 'Cassandra' from which Watson (1987) quotes: 'Why have women passion, intellect, moral activity – these three – and a place in society where no one of the three can be exercised?' Watson concludes:

Like the mythical Cassandra, Nightingale possessed the gift of prophecy and despaired at not being heard. The caring edge of nursing is dedicated to recreating the Cassandra myth by providing a place where the passion, intellect, and moral activity of women and nurses can be voiced and heard.

Cassandra was one of the daughters of the Greek mythical king Priam of Troy. 'The most common legend is that she was given the power of prophecy by Apollo, but was then doomed to be disbelieved because she refused him her love' (Radice, 1971, p. 83). Cassandra had tried to warn the Trojans against receiving the wooden horse, but was not listened to and Troy was destroyed. After the sacking of Troy she was murdered with Agamemnon, leader of the Greek forces in the Trojan war.

Cassandra has become the archetype of the woman who always speaks the truth and is never believed. Speaking the truth and having the power of prophecy go closely together. Prophecy is not 'foretelling' the future, but 'forthtelling' it by interpreting the signs of the times. By interpreting what is happening – speaking the truth – Cassandra became a prophet. The best-known prophets in the Judeo–Christian tradition, such as Isaiah and Jeremiah, had a very raw deal for speaking the truth based on their interpretations of what they saw happening around them.

If Florence Nightingale possessed the gift of prophecy like Cassandra, what does this say for nurses and nursing today? Do nurses still despair of not being able to exercise passion, intellect and moral activity? Do others see nurses as nourishers and healers, and nurses see themselves as ineffectual prophets, telling the truth and never being heard? This is certainly the impression one often gets. Florence Nightingale has become a model and for the general public – almost a mythical figure and idol. She is the lady with the lamp, the person who soothed heated brows, was always there when needed, never shirked any effort and went with the men into battles. But her legacy to her 'daughters' is that of a frustrated woman, passionate, intelligent, and asking of nurses the impossible in moral activity, if that means doing as she did. In this she has become a stereotype more than archetype. The archetype of the nurse, at least in Britain, is replaced by her stereotype. Is it possible, therefore, for nurses today to speak the truth as they interpret the signs of the times? Will they be heard any more than Cassandra was?

The truth today is that health care is in turmoil; resources are scarce; good nursing practice is eroded (Savage, 1995, p. 125); whistleblowers are silenced (Turner, 1992); and in government decisions nurses tend to be side-stepped (Carlisle, 1995).

The image of Cassandra, the woman who always tells the truth and is never taken seriously, fits the image of nursing well. Nightingale identified with this image, and seems to have experienced utter frustration in the role. The same can surely be said of many nurses today. Whatever truth they tell is not heard; whatever interpretation they make of the present is dismissed as either irrelevant or not correct. It seems that nurses are often listened to but never heard. Their words are heard, but the persons behind the words are not acknowledged. In order to remain persons of integrity under such circumstances, nurses either refuse to take on any responsibility beyond the actual job, or they leave the profession. Hitting against a brick wall becomes too painful after a certain time. Nightingale hit against the brick wall of the paternalism of Victorian England and the position of women in that culture. Today, nurses seem to hit the brick wall of the ideology of monetarism.

Whereas the archetype of the nurse as nurturer suits the individual better, the archetype of Cassandra seems to suit nursing as a whole more. Nursing as a profession seems to speak a truth without being heard. In this way the shadow of the archetype comes to the fore. While the archetypal nurse heals, comforts and nourishes, the shadow of the archetype withholds and refuses health. Nursing is not challenged into action by being sidelined: nursing seems to withdraw and even sulk. It is not fired into working towards new ways of healing and caring, but seems to slide into apathy and defence. Rather than finding the courage to adapt and change, nursing seems too often to be throwing up its arms in despair and let the world get on with its own affairs, not caring what happens to nursing. When the positive archetype is not able to function freely, the negative shadow makes itself felt all the more strongly until it takes over and then takes on a life of its own, being destructive.

Is there anything that can be done to change this state of affairs? What would fire nurses and nursing into action? What would help the positive archetype to establish itself again? Does nursing need its knight in shining armour to rescue it?

The symbol of the rescuer is a romantic idea which

cannot have a place in the present scenario. It is only in analysing and integrating its own archetype of mother and healer that nursing can be restored. Nursing has to nurse itself. By listening to its malaise, its sickness, and by hearing its wounds speak, nursing can take its rightful place again as the archetype it is. This is not a process which can be started at a conference or meeting. Giving attention to itself, mothering itself, nourishing itself, tending to itself, binding up its own wounds – all these are necessary. As nurses engage in this task, they will find that they meet many who also think and feel the same. One aspect of sickness is its loneliness, and when those who are sick and lonely get together (perhaps in a metaphorical Nightingale ward), then they can share and care for each other. When this happens, stories will be told – and above all heard.

♦

NURSING VALUES

Under this heading I do not want to rehearse the traditional values, but introduce some contradictions and opposites in order to examine the 'artistry' of nursing from some new angles, so that this idea of nursing caring for itself can be illuminated a little more.

Opposites

When considering nursing values, some opposites come quickly to mind (Table 4.1).

Much has been written about these values, both in theory and in practice. It is clear that the 'new' values need to be accepted, practised and integrated into care. Only in this way will they also be developed. The way in which patients and clients are nursed affects their well-being and recovery

♦ **Table 4.1** **Opposites in nursing values.**

Hierarchy	Democracy
Obedience	Initiative
Distance	Empathy
Extension	Expansion

The left-hand column represents traditional values and the right-hand column the values of the 'new nursing' (Savage, 1995).

significantly. This is not just an idealistic or extra dimension
to care, but affects also the economic state of any health care
in many different ways. Rather than look at these values as
such again, I want to suggest that they can also be
considered not so much as old and new in opposition, but as
valuable together in nursing at present and for the future.

Western psychology has attempted to access one opposite
pole and then the other (Wolinsky, 1994, p. 108), or to fuse
the opposites in a third point which then becomes
integration. But Wolinsky points out that this psychological
integration has never been really successful because polar
opposites are generally understood to be essentially different.

Wolinsky (1994) uses the insights and experiences of
physics – chaos theory in particular – to point to a different
way altogether. (Chaos theory maintains that 'apparently
random phenomena observed in various branches of science
result from complex dynamic underlying principles';
Chambers Dictionary, 1993.) Instead of concentrating on
opposites as being *different*, this theory sees opposites as
'being made of the same essential substance' (p. 108). When
opposites are seen to be made of the same substance, conflict
about them dissolves and the problem disappears. This, he
says, 'is true integration'. This may be a simple thing to say,
but to do it and live it is quite another matter. Wolinsky uses
many exercises to help his readers to understand this concept.

We spend much of our lives resisting the chaos which is
caused by opposites. If illness is the opposite of health, we
fight illness to get health back. If there is a shortage of
money, we work harder and harder to get money and thus
to restore the balance.

Some of the Eastern healing traditions, such as
acupuncture and shiatsu, use energy channels (meridians) to
restore health. When the meridian which connects with a
particular organ is stimulated at certain points, the energy is
freed to move again at the correct level and health can
return. By concentrating on the energy between health and
disease, these systems do not concentrate on opposites, but
on the flow between them. Essentially the same idea can be
applied to any problem. When this is done with the pairs of
opposites listed above, new patterns of energy begin to
emerge which may be interesting and revealing.

Instead of seeing one kind of value as old and therefore
outmoded and another value as new and therefore relevant
and better, seeing the energy which moves between them
also gives us energy. It is not only saying, 'the old still has

value', or 'we must respect a different tradition and culture', but it means an awareness of the energy which created the old and how this influences us still. The formation of the archetype of the nurse is made up of this energy. The shadow of the archetype, which resists, withholds and refuses, gains much of its validity from this image. There is a need to tap this energy and use it as part of an array of tactics available to nurses and nursing.

The new is only new when compared with the old. It grew out of a culture and situation (an energy) which had diminished and was therefore blocking progress. We create something new because we are essentially afraid of having nothing – emptiness or void – and are afraid of losing things and ourselves. Everything old disappears and we do not know what the new will be. Our efforts go therefore either into hanging on relentlessly to the old or into creating new things all the time in order to resist the chaos and emptiness which losing brings. The paradox is that we need to understand that everything changes, all the time. In other words, change is security; permanence is chaos. This gives a sense of freedom but makes us also vulnerable. Perhaps a 'new' value in nursing is vulnerability?

Wolinsky (1994, p. 107) says that:

> when spiritual or psychological systems begin to disappear back into emptiness they become more and more dogmatic and ritualised. This dogmatic and ritualistic tendency is a survival mechanism of ... any hierarchy.

Hierarchy vs. democracy

A hierarchical authority in nursing is therefore not something which is old and old-fashioned, but a present energy 'packet' (or quantum) which is maintained in order to resist the chaos created by democracy. Democracy is not so much the opposite of authority, but both are part of a constantly changing system. It is not so much that democracy is better than authority, but that we are afraid of the chaos caused by the change which either system brings; therefore we go with the safety of the known system. Dare we, as individuals and as professionals, go with the vulnerability of the change?

In a hierarchically authoritarian system a great deal of emphasis is placed on obedience, and on belief and faith rather than on present experience. But to say that democracy is better and ought therefore to be practised is not necessarily right either. Democracy is certainly the system which is better suited to today's health care scene as it takes into consideration the personal and collective rights and responsibilities which go with that system. The question may not be that we fight for one system or another, but that we experience the energy of the system which is most appropriate for the present, and dissipate that energy, knowing that the system does and will change.

Obedience vs. initiative

The idea that nurses are 'seen but not heard' had its day and place in the past. Today, nurses make it a virtue to be seen and heard. Not only is the virtue of obedience rejected, but independence is stressed. This is an independence of spirit, mind and professional knowledge. It is made obvious in the kind of imaginative relationships which are enjoyed and stressed not just in nursing. Telling stories has become an accepted form of teaching and learning. There need not be anything extraordinary about the story; on the contrary, it may be some very small event which is related but which becomes important in the telling of it. It takes imagination to see that the ordinary is also extraordinary. What matters is that initiative was recognized, both in the self and in others.

When nurses were 'neither maid nor nun' (as the title of a recent exhibition at the International Red Cross in Geneva, Switzerland, portrayed nurses), their place was at the beck and call of others, usually doctors. Serving others gave them little room for personal development and independence which might have been expressed in initiative.

But while nurses are no longer the doctors' handmaidens, it seems they have now become the employers' handmaidens. A contract offered to a staff nurse by a trust hospital states: 'In the course of your normal work with the trust you will come into possession of confidential information concerning patients, the trust and its staff. Such information must always be treated as strictly confidential and further must not be divulged to any individual or organisation, including the press, without prior written approval by the chief executive or his (sic) nominated deputy' (personal communication).

Clearly, nursing is not free of the subservient role. The difference is that in the past nurses would not have thought twice about such a contract; today, rightly, they not only question it but also question its legitimacy. But today also, the opposition is much stronger and tougher and nurses are more easily pushed into corners where exploitation and abuse of powers are possible. Is it therefore not a matter of both obedience and initiative being used together? The person who uses initiative in relation to a client, patient or chief executive needs a high degree of commitment, which can also be expressed as obedience to a value which stems originally from the principle to respect the person. This means oneself in the first instance, and others by extension.

Distance vs. empathy

Not so long ago individual nurses were helped to 'avoid the experience of anxiety, guilt, doubt and uncertainty' (Menzies, 1960). Today, 'engrossment' (Noddings, 1984, p. 74) and 'involvement' (Savage, 1995, p. 1) are the means of being empathic. In the way which I am suggesting here, perhaps the two elements are not simply opposites but part of the same concept.

One element of empathy is to keep one foot on firm ground while helping the client or patient out of the present ditch (Tschudin, 1995, p. 77). For empathy to function therefore, there has to be a degree of detachment. Many ethicists would say that moral reasoning and objectivity are the only bases on which to make good decisions. This demands a high degree of detachment from the persons concerned. It must at least be questionable if this is really possible.

Menzies suggested that nurses constantly were 'involved' with their patients and wanted to be, but that their system of management saw to it that the psychological 'remnants' (shadows) which management could not or would not face, were never tapped. This meant that there was a great deal of suffering for nurses which was dealt with either by leaving training, seeking postgraduate training, or by being sick. By stressing empathy today, nursing has taken a great step forward in assuring a psychologically healthier work force. But do nurses really understand the ingredients and implications of empathy?

Mayeroff (1971, p. 11) lists 'alternating rhythms' as one of the 'major ingredients of caring' which he describes. He says that in caring for a person 'there are times when I do not inject myself into the situation, I do not take a stand one way or the other, I do 'nothing'. And when I undergo this "inactivity", I see what resulted from it and [I] may change my behaviour accordingly'. Distance and empathy need not be opposites but the two sides of the same coin. Distance has its limits and empathy has its limits; distance is needed and empathy is needed for a relationship (particularly a helping relationship) to be healthy.

Extension vs. expansion

According to Mackay (1993, p. 240), extending the role of nurses is a 'strategy which the nursing profession has used to overcome the imbalances in the doctor–nurse relationship' in order 'to define the division of labour between nurses and doctors'. Extension means basically that nurses can carry out certain tasks which before were the duties of the medical profession, such as 'the administration of intravenous drugs, taking blood samples, doing ECGs (electrocardiograms). This is 'elongating specific, already assumed functions' (Zornow, 1977, in Pearson, 1983, p. 12), whereas 'expansion is a fundamentally different concept ... concerned with a "deepening" and development of the role, drawing on those skills and areas of knowledge which are uniquely nursing' (Pearson, 1983, p. 12). Extension follows a medical model; expansion develops a nursing model.

This division has been recognized by the UKCC in its *Scope of Professional Practice* (1992b) which states (paragraph 13) that 'a concentration of "activities" can detract from the importance of holistic nursing care'. Nevertheless, nurses have to (and presumably enjoy having to) take on tasks which give them a sense and image of technical ability. Increasingly, nurses also have to take on tasks of management, being in charge of ward and departmental budgets and having to negotiate contracts for purchaser and provider services.

The division between extension and expansion is perhaps the most significant among the opposites considered here. Extension is along horizontal lines and expansion along vertical lines, thus going in opposite directions. Yet, both movements are necessary. Nurses may be very torn in their loyalties if they have to choose between the one or the other. But can they combine the two?

I have considered the other pairs of opposites as part of the same essential substance; another dimension or symbol comes to light here. When vertical and horizontal meet, they form a cross. This crossing over and meeting happens in the present, and in the person who experiences tension or chaos. It can therefore be said more clearly than before, that in the very fact of constantly adjusting, considering the other person or aspect, and experiencing the tension, lies the security which is needed in order to be alive and keep alive.

If this was perhaps more an exercise in psychology and physics, where is the morality of it? Niebuhr (1963, p. 56) suggests that in order to be and remain human, we *respond*. First of all we are people, engaged in dialogue, acting in response to actions upon us. This ability to respond leads to responsibility. We understand ourselves as 'responsive beings' which leads us towards both goal seeking and respect for the law. In themselves the pursuit of goals (portrayed by the symbol of 'the maker') or the keeping of laws (portrayed by the symbol of 'the citizen') are usually considered to be opposites in ethical theories. Responsibility (using the symbol of 'the answerer') is not only an alternative way, but a way which goes deeper and further. It goes deeper in that it starts with the person who is a moral agent; and it goes further in that it does not stop at either a goal or a law, but seeks a 'social solidarity' beyond either goal or law.

In experiencing the present, that is, being aware, hearing, giving attention, we tap into the energy which each person and thing has and gives. When we are aware we are also responsible; when we are responsible we are also aware. This is perhaps the basic moral stance to ourselves and to others. In order to be responsible we have to know many things. Images, opposites, symbols, meanings and interpretations are just part of this basic knowing which is expressed in responsibility.

◆

MATTERING

I am using the expression 'mattering' in the way Oppenheimer (1995) described it at a conference and subsequently in print. Oppenheimer is a philosopher and theologian who has not lost 'the common touch'; her paper is full of such everyday things as roses, curved cucumbers, children's teddy bears, slugs and cakes. She says 'people matter; mattering matters; and mattering is more given than chosen'.

The principle that *people matter*, Oppenheimer believes,

is a great improvement on 'respect for persons'. She asks, 'Human beings seem to be given responsibility by their Creator to create other persons: but how far does this responsibility extend?' This is a crucial question for nurses who '*must*', in the exercise of professional accountability, 'promote and safeguard the interests and well-being of patients and clients' (UKCC, 1992a). Does responsibility for nurses extend into 'creating' persons? When we create good environments, good teams, good practices, is this enough? Are nurses also responsible for ensuring that patients are emotionally well cared for, can be creative and adapt well to the present circumstances?

Oppenheimer says that a person can be defined as a 'pattern of lovability'. Many nurses find very little lovability in patients, particularly 'not nice, old, male patients' (Greipp, 1996). Even an unlovable person still matters. This may be one way in which we can start to care without having to do mental gymnastics to come to the same conclusion.

'To say that *mattering matters* is to use 'mattering' as a bridge between fact and value', says Oppenheimer. She also uses the term 'minding' as a bridge. Minding is not an abstract mental activity, but minding is also caring. People mind (care) and therefore they matter. Caring is the basic human mode of being (Roach, 1992, p. xi). Caring is not just an instinct but is that which makes a person human. Caring is therefore also the basic moral act. Facts are not 'value-free' but have value, as it were, built into them. Facts and values are another pair of opposites which may be seen to be of the same substance when that substance – mattering – is the energy which binds them together.

Nurses are on the whole great diplomats, able to interpret a doctor's language to a patient, and a patient's language to a doctor; they are able to judge what a patient needs and then tell a doctor in such a way that the doctor makes the (right) decision. They are first class bridge builders in these activities. When they show that mattering matters, their care is moral.

The question of the nature of values is addressed by the statement that *mattering is more given than chosen*. Oppenheimer says that 'we have a lot of control over facts, but values are given to us'. She writes about life-styles being a choice but says that mattering goes further. She calls herself an 'intuitionist', 'if that means that I think of values as findable by something like looking'. The values one finds depend on the choice one makes by taking a particular stance. A house is bigger when observed from close up than from a distance. But things matter in relation to people: 'the mattering of people cannot be separated from the interconnectedness of their minding'.

An ultimate question (which Oppenheimer asks at the end of her paper) is, how different values and different life-styles can be fitted together into a system which is integrated and coherent. With many insoluble problems about priorities, she suggests that some of the hardest problems are practical rather than theoretical. She says that both a drunken tramp and Michelangelo matter and if they are both in a burning building 'we are in great trouble'. Nurses know this trouble well – only too well in today's climate of scarce resources of people, money and goods. Oppenheimer tries to answer her own question in terms of the traditional ultimate values of truth, beauty and goodness.

She says that there are moral truths as well as factual truths and gives some examples from literature. The same can be attempted by using the examples of the archetypes of the nurse and of Cassandra. There is no doubt about the moral truth of nurses: they nurture, help, relieve, heal and cherish. In this way they encourage and empower their clients and patients to health and recovery or to a peaceful death. This is also true of the archetypal nurses: they do the same but at a different level. The truth is the same (as Cassandra maintained); the facts and the values may change. It may not be a question of integrating the differences so much as seeing opposites here, too, not as polarities, but as part of the same essence.

When it comes to goodness and beauty, Oppenheimer suggests that the principle 'people matter' is 'a first step towards fitting creativity into the same system as moral goodness'. Minding is

> the basis of people's mattering to themselves, to one another, and to God. The whole area we so inadequately call 'aesthetic' comes in when we go on to ask what there is for them to mind about. Instead of 'minding' we can say 'loving'. ... As soon as we give love something to do we open the way to other valid concerns besides being good.

We are not 'good' for our own ends but in order to create a society – a heaven – where people do not just sit around playing harps but where people grow by doing real things. The 'good life' is not only the after-life, but this life in which beauty, the aesthetic and pleasure are its substance. 'Then we might say that goodness is its form; and truth, that is, reality, its condition'.

It is often difficult for nurses to think of nursing in terms of 'love'. Love is an emotive word which cannot be applied to a job. It may be possible for some nurses, perhaps those working in paediatric care, to say that they do a lot of loving, but the same cannot be said of nurses in A&E or in operating theatres. Indeed, in these areas of care, detachment is more appropriate. Perhaps it can be said here, too, that attachment and detachment are not opposites, but part of the same continuum. What we do as people cannot ever adequately be described; sooner or later we reach an end with words and concepts and love is the only means of describing that which we do to others.

I believe that what Oppenheimer is trying to express is what many before her have been trying to express eloquently, and what every nurse tries to express, more or less eloquently, and certainly practically, is the search for what makes us human; what it means to be human; and how this is expressed. Trying to answer this will lead us to others as well as away from them. We are attracted as well as revolted by others. We are ourselves attractive to some and revolting to others. When all is said and done, many of us will say with St Augustine 'Love, and do as you will'. What matters is that we are not afraid of loving, whatever 'loving' means.

♦

THE MORAL ART

The concept which frames a great deal of contemporary academic discussion is that of 'post-modernism'. It is claimed by some that this is characterised by a move away from grand theories and beliefs in overarching solutions towards a more pragmatic flexibility which allows for a variety of perspectives. It can be found across the whole field of human endeavour; in art, architecture, medicine, science, technology and politics.

(Horton, Bayne and Bimrose, 1995)

Is nursing also, in the post-modern world, moving towards pragmatic flexibility and new perspectives? Certainly the issues raised by Oppenheimer as 'mattering' are one effort to address the pragmatism needed in an effort to go forward morally.

In this last section I shall examine a number of topics which all relate to moral artistry but from diverse angles and positions, and consider them in the light of some of the foregoing ideas.

Caring and curing

Watson (1988) writes about caring and curing, but not in the sense of medicine doing the curing and nursing the caring. She says that 'the future of medicine *and* [emphasis added] nursing belongs to *caring* more than *curing*. ... (T)here is a movement out of an era in which *curing* is dominant into an era in which *caring* must take precedence'.

Gadow in Watson and Ray (1988, p. 6) describes the inverted relationship between cure and care by

> ... designating care as the highest form of commitment to patients, encompassing as many different expressions of concern for patient well-being as we are imaginative enough to devise; the frustrating situations will be those in which the scope of our concern is limited to a single treatable problem, in the care for which there is nothing to do but provide the remedy. There is, in other words, *nothing but cure* that we can offer, if the situation is so constricted that the infinitely more encompassing breath of care either cannot be offered or received.

This is an interesting example of two polarities which have changed place. If this is indeed possible, does it not show that they are part of the same continuum and in fact part of the same substance? It is not so much a swing to the opposite pole, as care and cure being part of the same means of responding to a person in need. This response is the most fitting for that particular person at that time in those circumstances. The interesting thing is that for most other people in similar circumstances care is now becoming the fitting response. This change has come about for various reasons, the main one being that people are more and more aware of their personal needs which had been suppressed in favour of technology and science. Perhaps one of the hallmarks of post-modern society is that it can say that just because machines and cures are available, we do not need to use them. This shows a new independence of mind and body which is ready enough to be vulnerable. It shows also that by going along with the essential energy in the person – and the culture and community – the fitting response will be found and is acceptable.

It will be interesting to see if caring will become the dominant aspect of health care and how it will happen. What is clear is that cure is increasingly ruining societies and nations financially.

Caring too much and not caring enough

Quinn (1994, p. 64) writes about caring too much and not caring enough. The nurses she works with do not complain that they have to care too much, but that in fact they are not permitted to care in the systems in which they work. Quinn sees this as being similar to a phenomenon known among the shamans or healers. The shamans are 'called' to be healers, usually in a prophetic dream. When the person does not follow the call, serious and even fatal illness will ensue. This can be physical or mental illness, leading possibly to psychosis. Quinn believes that this is 'essentially the manifestation of inner despair and turmoil created by the failure to follow the call of one's heart'.

The shadow of the nurse – the withholder of healing and nourishment – is possibly also a manifestation of such a sickness. When a nurse cannot care or is not permitted to care by the system, then the shadow grows longer and longer over the soul and consciously or unconsciously negative power is exerted. This may, as in this case, be a defence, and once the nurse is again in a position to care, this shadow disappears. When the un-caring goes on without relief, then sickness or psychosis will almost inevitably manifest itself, usually as 'burnout'.

It would seem very important therefore that nurses and nursing take the prophetic role seriously and become more and more aware of the need to care for themselves and for others, as only in that way can humans as people and humanity itself be healed. Nurses are still 'called' to exercise their prophetic role. Indeed if they do not fulfil their role, then they can be sidelined. This 'call' is nothing mystical (in the sense of secretive), but is the basic challenge to each professional to act in the most authentic way possible. This is also the most moral way, if we like it or not. To act less than morally is also to act less than fully effectively as persons and professionals. This is the ideal; clearly there are times and places when this is not possible, and good is not done, the best is not available and the negative energy wins. The 'problem of evil' cannot be brushed aside; it is also part of the continuum. Morality and ethics are to do with the way in which we deal with it.

Private life and professional persona

This leads me to consider the dichotomy which seems to exist between private life and professional persona. A friend put it to me thus:

> I am really bothered that nursing – and nursing ethics – is sometimes portrayed as something separate – as if there is a value system underpinning our personal lives and a separate value system underpinning our work as nurses. Maybe it is something about bringing our selves into our care so that the 'me' outside the uniform (and the values underpinning 'me') is the same 'me' as when I am in uniform.

It seems that 'nursing as a moral art' is precisely this 'bringing our selves into our care' in a way which does not diminish the essential 'me' and yet does not overstretch the professional 'me' either. How does one learn this, let alone teach it? Scott (1995) argues that 'students and practitioners (should be) facilitated in developing an ethical awareness and sensitivity from early in their professional development'. This does not mean that studying how sensitivity develops makes one sensitive.

Nurses have traditionally learned by observation and repetitive practice. This is not too difficult when it concerns manual and psychomotor skills, but are virtues learned by 'sitting by Nellie'?

When ethics first came on the scene in nursing it was clearly principles oriented, and mainly based on the model of medical ethics. This is beginning to be questioned. Nurses are struggling with other ways of expressing their essential 'me' which is more adequate and more holistic (Scott, 1995; Begley, 1995; James, 1995; Oberle, 1995). This is far from easy, as indeed Oppenheimer (1995) above has also demonstrated. The language is difficult, clumsy even. We use old-fashioned words and give them new meaning because we have no modern words. We talk about virtues (which seems to be linked to Victorian values) and morality (which usually meant either religion or sexuality) and calling (which was also about religion).

What all this points to is that the experience itself matters again to people. Principles are abstract things which can be applied to some big issues, such as euthanasia or abortion (Hanford, 1993), and if we knew how to do this in the right way, we would be considered ethical. Nurses are rightly not satisfied with this approach because they deal with many more issues every day which are just as important as euthanasia or abortion but which have never been discussed in textbooks. If they are not in the textbooks, nurses do not know how to face them, hence the dichotomy between private and professional values. When there is no professional value basis for most of the situations in which nurses find themselves, can they allow or trust their private values to influence or professional practice? And vice versa?

In this chapter I have tried to show that the personal influences the professional, and the professional influences the private all along. If they are seen as opposites, they clash, but if they are seen as part of the same substance, then there may be less of a problem. The opposites come together in our selves; this is where the experience takes place. This is therefore also the 'place' where the awareness is, where the decision is made and where the consequences are experienced. The consequences are too often a guilt at not having acted with integrity and anger at having been put in situations where one's 'calling' or caring was not possible. The 'answer' lies not in splitting the personal from the professional, but in being more aware of and more sensitive to the present situation. This is where the chaos and the vulnerability are; it is also where the energy is.

Responsibility

If withdrawal is not the answer, then responsibility must be considered as the more likely promising answer. This means both a personal and a professional involvement.

May (1994) writes that

> Moral reflection ... does not simply trace back to a brace of sometimes conflicting principles; it forces

meditation on the human condition; it probes one's deepest convictions; it may even unsettle one's habits; it asks of the agent the mobilisation of resources, some of them already in place but untested; others, as yet, unbidden.

The *a*bility to respond (Niebuhr, 1963, p. 57) leads to respons*i*bility, that is, the personal ability leads to attitudes and actions related to others.

Medical ethics, and in particular the principles mostly associated with it – autonomy, beneficence, nonmaleficence, justice – have 'failed to pursue with sufficient imagination the idea of the common good' (Callahan, 1994) because they have tended 'to reduce the problem of the common good to justice, and the individual moral life to the gaining of autonomy'. In doing so, personal responsibility and the moral use of personal choice have been sidelined. An ethic of personal responsibility leads to a communitarian ethic. Niebuhr (1963, p. 65) is clear that personal responsibility leads to 'social solidarity'. As we respond to others, they respond to us, and so on in continuing interactions. This continuity forms one personally and forms a community of moral agents. Responsibility is thus a movement from 'I' to 'we' and back again. In this movement is the energy which combines the opposites of I and we, singular and plural, personal good and common good.

This responsibility is perhaps above all an awareness of the impact we have on others. In terms of ethics this means being aware of the other or others. Being aware is a long way away from doing what they want. But then ethics is not simply responding to what they (or I) want – or assuring that there is a choice – but making the kind of choices which are relevant to the community, that is, to all of us.

Attention, compassion, forgiveness

In a small book entitled *The Power of Compassion* the Dalai Lama (1995) writes a great deal about affection (or warm-heartedness), compassion and forgiveness. He stresses also the use of meditation. Since some of the concepts above about opposites and sameness are essentially Eastern in origin, awareness which I have mentioned often, and the stress on meditation all have to do with basic attention, I propose here to put this word together with compassion and forgiveness.

To experience a situation or a challenge fully is often quite difficult. We experience ourselves, but not the other person also, or the wider implications. After the event most of us can be wise, say the right thing, have the right reaction, but in the event itself this is a different matter. Giving attention to ourselves, to others and to events demands a great deal of training and willpower. When we can be attentive we know how good and empowering it is.

Giving clear attention is also difficult for most people because as soon as we are aware of something, we judge it. 'I should not have said that', or 'I can never get what I want' are just two of the types of judgements we make all day when we become aware. A non-judgmental attitude is one of the pre-conditions often used in counselling. There it means not judging the other person. But how can we be non-judgmental with others if we cannot be so with ourselves? Giving attention to ourselves in a non-judgmental way is therefore a fundamental basis for being with others.

'Compassion' says the Dalai Lama (p.74) 'is the key factor for all human business'. His idea of compassion ranges very widely from religious practice to the question of the future of humanity, the complexity and inter-connectedness of the nature of modern existence, and no longer feeling indifferent or dismissing them when we think of 'others'.

Compassion is also something which we show towards ourselves. When we are judgmental towards ourselves we are not compassionate towards ourselves; when we become non-judgmental we also become compassionate. I said above that any profession has to be first to itself what it would do to others. So nurses have to be nurses to themselves first if they are to be true nurses to others. This becomes clear in this exploration about compassion. Nurses are not nurses only for the hours when they wear a uniform or are on duty. We bear the archetype of the nurse and that means caring for ourselves, being compassionate to ourselves, nourishing ourselves, healing ourselves. This is not a self-seeking activity, but a basic human necessity. In responding to ourselves in this way we learn how to respond to those with whom we are in community.

Forgiveness is a religious act, deliberately sought and given. It is also a very human act. Psychiatrists probably call it 'letting go'. In the image used in this chapter, it could also apply to accepting the idea of chaos, going with the energy rather than against it, thus possessing the only worthwhile and sure knowledge.

In my work as a counsellor I find that these three elements are absolutely basic. Each is as difficult as the other. Paying attention to some aspect of the person can be very painful. I often ask patients to 'sit' with something, perhaps anger, fear or some image from the past. This is not easy because in our world we are used to being able to have things fixed and pain removed quickly. When this sitting or meditating can be done, most people find that it is this which will have led them further. The sitting-with is a kind of compassion to oneself: caring deeply, not judging, not taking over, but not standing by idle either. When the feeling, memory or pain has been considered in this compassionate way, then it will eventually lose its power and that is when the forgiveness comes. The thing which has terrorized oneself perhaps for long years loses its power when faced. Then it can be seen for what it is really: an outdated defence or a bogey from the past. It can be laid to rest now, forgiven and let go of.

Attention, compassion and forgiveness are perhaps not words which are daily on the lips of nurses, but they are attitudes and values which are basic to moral beings. One way of bridging the gap between the personal 'me' and the professional 'me' is to see that these basic elements apply to both sides and that in applying them from both standpoints, the difference between personal and professional disappears.

In the way we deal with ourselves we deal also with other people, such as clients, patients and colleagues. When we experience attention, compassion and forgiveness with and to ourselves, we can also apply them to others. We have the choice to do it; the moral 'art' is how we do it.

Political awareness

If we take seriously the idea that caring is the future of all health care, then all the points just made are part of that care. It is not *that* we care which is moral, but *how* we care. Condon (1992) writes that 'the moral quality of caring in nursing emerges from the idea of commitment to a particular end ... the protection and enhancement of human dignity'.

The kind of caring which Watson (1989) describes will need to be accompanied by an ethic of caring. Establishing such an ethic of caring

that avoids features of oppression and exploitation will ... depend on the emergence of caring as a political

> philosophy capable of transforming institutions and
> the politics within which nursing is practised, on
> removing bureaucratic barriers to caring practice, and
> on removing conditions that exploit nurses in the carer
> role
>
> (Condon, 1992).

The word 'political' strikes fear into many nurses' hearts. A decade or so ago, nurses tended to say 'don't bother me with ethics, just let me get on with caring'; but they had to learn about ethics in order to care. Now the cry is perhaps 'I don't want to be political; I just want to care'. We may soon all have to take courses in politics in order to care effectively. The sense in which the word is used here has not to do with party-political activity, but with its root sense: the Greek *polites* meaning citizen.

If caring is about the protection and enhancement of human dignity, then it matters crucially what we mean by human dignity. Many of the issues considered in this chapter have tried to address this topic. The fact that the NHS is built on a philosophy of care for all regardless of ability to pay has perhaps given nurses a false sense of justice. We assume that equality exists when and where it does not. The stance of patient advocate is becoming more and more important in nursing and is indeed a political stance. When acting as advocates, nurses challenge inequality, injustice, indignity and the lapses and reductions of dignity. This is not only on a directly patient-centred level, but also on the level of policies and administration. Albarran (1995) says that

> The UKCC implies that a nurse's duty must be to act
> and, when necessary, stress the shortcomings of health
> care policies in the institution or the community, which
> may also be perceived as political advocacy. ... From
> this stance, the duty of care demands a duty to be
> politically responsive.

In an ethic of care (Watson, 1989) and a politics of care (Tronto, 1993, p. 172) there is a strong emphasis on democracy, mutuality and reciprocity. This implies that there is a great deal of listening (Tronto, 1993, p. 172), attending (above), receptivity, relatedness and responsiveness (Noddings, 1984, p. 2), attitudes and actions directed toward specific people rather than systems (Condon, 1992) and fostering growth in one another (Bergum, 1994). These elements are not just beneficial for patients and clients, but, because the caring relationship is central, they 'would tend to limit if not eliminate exploitation or oppression of the carer at least at the level of the individual if not at the bureaucratic level (Condon, 1992). When there is no exploitation, either of the patient by the carer, or the carer by the bureaucracy, then caring is really happening.

When there is exploitation there is always a top-dog and an under-dog: another example of polar opposites, only in this instance it is not some abstract like day and night, but it touches people in their essential humanity. The fact that essays like this one are written points to the need, not so much to give a balance, as to highlight where the energy is and to restore the right or fitting level of energy.

By working towards an elimination of exploitation and oppression of the cared-for and the carers, and protecting and enhancing human dignity, nurses already have a political role, whether they want to or not, or are aware of it or not. When they are not aware of it the shadow of the nurse can swing powerfully into action, exploiting and oppressing patients.

Perhaps the moral art of nursing is to become what it truly is already: nursing.

♦

CONCLUSION I started this chapter by perversely asking if *nursing* can be moral rather than individual nurses. This needs to be addressed again now. What one person does inevitably reflects on the group to which this person belongs. One rotten apple in a basket full of apples quickly affects them all. When all the apples are good, there is no danger of going bad. But nature – agricultural or human – is not perfect. If it were, there would be no growth, understanding or choice possible. Thank God, then, for imperfection. Or is this perverse, too? Because there is not just imperfection, but evil, suffering and pain which are infinitely worse than imperfection. After all, a bad apple can and does affect a whole basket full of apples: they all go rotten. Reinhold Niebuhr, the brother of the author I cited most on responsibility, wrote a book with the title *Moral Man and Immoral Society* (1932). Can one remain moral when all around are immoral, and without becoming angry?

This is perhaps too big a question for most of us. After all, our sphere of influence is generally quite small. The real question may be, do most of us use all the space of the sphere of influence we have? Who are we moral to and with?

By considering some not-so-obvious aspects of nursing, such as the archetypes, the role of prophecy in nursing, and old and new values and putting them under a different light (energy) I have tried to address some aspects of morality. Generally, morality is understood to be referring to a private sphere and that which one does mostly at home with the doors closed: one's private practice of religion or sexuality.

By the mere fact that we are human beings, we have to relate to others. This relating may be more or less obvious, or more or less easy. In whatever way we relate, it calls for wider responses: memories, fantasies, feelings are deeply involved in every kind of short and long encounter. We can choose to attend or not, and how we attend. If you as a patient or client smile at me or I as a nurse hit you, this has much to do with nature and nurture, memories, ideals, energy, past and present values and experiences, state of health and will. It has also to do with being an individual citizen who is also a professional nurse. I cannot be judged only on one aspect.

Having considered some ideas of opposites not being seen as opposites but as part of a continuing whole, I would like to end with the alchemical proverb 'As above, so below'. The alchemists had tried to transmute other metals into gold, and to discover the elixir of life. At the level of the purely physical they failed, but their understanding of the integration of opposites has never been questioned. So it is possible to say also, as inside, so outside; as one, so all; as all, so one. What nurses are personally, nursing as a profession is. This has its positive side and its negative, its good and its bad, its constructive and destructive, its exciting and its hampering. But perhaps they are not opposites, but part of the whole idea and reality which, when seen with your ears and heard with your eyes become an art, and a moral art.

Conversation

CHAPTER 5   *You seem to have moved well away from the sorts of things nurses usually write about. The theory–practice gap is a more familiar topic when reading exposition on the science and art of nursing.*

CHAPTER 4   *The problem with that view is that it focuses on old thinking where opposites are in conflict with each other. I have shown that opposites are connected, like the faces of a cube.*

CHAPTER 5   *That came over strongly to me. Now I can come back to some of the ideas from philosophy which Chapters 1 and 2 talked about. I want to show how intuition has got lost along the way, in favour of other forms of knowledge.*

CHAPTER 4   *I think nurses must practise responsibly, according to their values.*

CHAPTER 5   *Yes, that's true, and I will suggest that as well as values, the decisions nurses make emerge from many forms of knowledge, including intuition....*

INTUITION: 'JUST KNOWING' IN NURSING

Diane Marks-Maran

It was 02.15 in the morning. The setting, a large teaching hospital. I was sister in charge of a group of six wards on that particular night. As I was beginning my rounds of visits to my wards, I suddenly heard my 'bleep.' I went to the nearest telephone to respond. It was the senior staff nurse on one of my six wards. The conversation between her and myself went something like this:

ME   Hello staff nurse. You bleeped me. What can I do for you?
STAFF NURSE I am worried about Mrs Janes, the lady with ischaemic heart disease. Her observations are stable – pulse is 70, blood pressure is 140/60 but I just know that something isn't quite right...

ME   OK, I'm on my way.

I went straight to the ward and arrived just in time to see the resuscitation team racing into the ward. Mrs Janes had suffered a cardiac arrest.

  This is not a unique story, but it is a true one. How did the staff nurse know? What had she observed or sensed or felt or thought? Was it coincidence, prior experience, or was it intuition?

  This chapter will attempt to explore intuition in nursing, its legitimacy and its place in clinical judgement and practice. The chapter will begin with a brief look at some of the philosophical history contributing to the debate about knowledge, reasoning, sensing and science. Intuition will then be comprehensively explained and defined. The place of intuition in science and in art will also be examined. Finally, I will put forward an argument for wisdom in nursing, using the theory of psychological types of Jung (1875–1961) and relate Jung's four mental processes: sensing, intuition, feeling and thinking, as a framework for exploring what nursing wisdom might be.

◆

FROM WHENCE WE COME

Throughout history philosophers have argued and counter-argued about concepts like sensing, reasoning, knowledge and intuition. Plato, (c. 427–347 BC), for example, believed that the highest degree of reality is that which we think with our reason. Aristotle (384–322 BC), on the other hand, believed that the highest degree of reality is that which we perceive with our senses. Who is right? In fact, it doesn't matter. Each represents a different paradigm or world view, a different face on the cube, about knowledge and where it comes from. Thus was born the dualism between sensing and reasoning, a dualism which is still argued today. Aristotle believed that there was nothing in our consciousness except that which we have first experienced with our senses. All our thoughts and ideas come into our consciousness through that which we have seen, heard or felt. All human beings, according to Aristotle, have an innate ability to take all sensory experiences and organize them into categories. Human beings, therefore, have no innate ideas; they only have the inborn ability to reason. This ability to reason, however, is empty or inert until such time as we experience something through our senses. It is then that our reasoning gives meaning to our sensory experiences.

As we move into the Middle Ages there was a general belief in the European scholarly communities of that time that all problems in the world could be solved purely by thought and reasoning. However, the Renaissance heralded a change in scholarly thinking away from blind adherence to rationality (reason) and towards a belief that phenomena in the world should use the investigative processes of the senses. The rise of empiricism – investigation by observation, experience and experiment – was a feature of this time. Without this new paradigm shift or changing world view, all the technical advances of the Renaissance would not have happened.

This new empirical method was based on the then new belief that we can only base our knowledge on our experiences. Experimental methodology and method became the primary sources of legitimate knowledge. This paved the way for a fundamental breakthrough in philosophy. Human beings broke away from the notion that they were merely a part of nature. Bacon (1561–1626), an English philosopher of the time expressed this change when he said that knowledge is power. Two new notions were embedded in this short phrase: firstly, that knowledge has a practical value and, secondly, that human beings could influence nature, or even control it.

The concept of scientific method was born in the new philosophic approach to knowledge in the Renaissance, a method which was a direct result of the paradigm shift at the time away from investigation, using reason and thinking towards investigation by observation, experience and experiment. Having said all this, it would be wrong to paint a picture of the Renaissance as an era of organized thinking despite the fact that it brought us scientific method. Despite the new ideas in the Renaissance about knowledge and the resulting technological and scientific advantages, it was still a time of disorganized thought and understanding. It was a mixture of old beliefs and thinking and new beliefs and thinking – about nature, science, knowledge, god and humanity.

In the 17th century Descartes (1596–1650), a French philosopher, suggested that we cannot accept anything as true unless we can clearly perceive it. He was seeking a method by which human beings could be certain about the nature of life. To do this, he found it necessary to begin by doubting and questioning all that he had learned up until that time to 'rid himself of all handed down or received learning before beginning his own philosophical construction' (Gaarder, 1995, p. 183). He even proposed that he should doubt all that his senses told him suggesting that it was possible that even they were deceiving him.

In setting himself this enormous task of doubting all previous learning and all sensory experiences, he came to realize that the only one certainty in life is doubt. When he doubted, he was thinking and, because he was thinking, it had to be true that he was a thinking being. He expressed this realization in his famous quote, '*Cognito ergo sum*' (I think, therefore I am). In many respects this revelation experienced by Descartes was an intuitive experience yet he, like the philosophers of the Middle Ages, was a rationalist. He believed in reason as the primary source of knowledge. One could speculate that Descartes found the roots of his own rationalism through an intuitive event. His ultimate goal was to arrive at ultimate knowledge based on reasoning.

In the 18th century rationalism as the primary source of legitimate knowledge began to be seriously questioned and criticized. The philosophical writings of the time, primarily in Britain, began to return to Aristotle's belief that there is nothing in the mind which has not first been perceived in the senses. This began the rise of empiricism – those who saw all of knowledge coming from that which our senses told us.

Empiricists believe (and argue) that human beings are not born with ideas and that any idea which cannot be related to sensory experience must be a false idea. The consuming work of many of the 18th century empiricists was to scrutinize all human ideas and concepts to see if there was any basis for them in actual experience. Locke (1632–1704), for example, who was one of the 18th century British empiricists, examined two fundamental questions about knowledge: from where do we get our ideas? Can we rely on our senses and experiences? He created the notion of 'simple ideas of sense' which can be explained thus: as a person senses or experiences something from outside, this sensation (experience) enters the mind as an idea. The mind works on the idea – by thinking, reasoning, classifying, doubting, believing, questioning – a series of processes which Locke called *reflection*. Locke, therefore, differentiates between sensing and reflecting. All complex ideas can be traced back to 'simple ideas of sense' – taste, smell, colour, sound. Knowledge which cannot be traced back to these 'simple ideas of sense' must be false knowledge and should, therefore, be rejected.

This was how Locke came to answer the first of his questions. With regard to his second question, 'Can we rely on what our senses tell us?', he suggests that sensation has two qualities – primary qualities and secondary qualities. Primary qualities were things we sensed which were measured or quantifiable (height, weight, speed, amount) and we could, therefore, be confident that our senses reproduced them accurately. Secondary qualities of sensation, however, are those sensations like taste, smell, sound or colour which were qualitative. We do not perceive the real qualities of these sensations; we only perceive the effect they have upon us. We can *think* that a primary quality is what it is but we can only *believe* a secondary quality. Locke therefore agreed with Descartes, that reality contains certain qualities that human beings are able to understand through reason.

The 19th century saw a number of philosophical paradigm shifts. Two which are worthy of note are positivism and existentialism. Positivism had its roots in the empirical movement of the previous century. Comte (1789–1857), a French philosopher in the 19th century, was one of the foremost positivist philosophers of science. Positivism argues that scientists search for objective knowledge which is able to explain phenomena as well as to predict and control how those phenomena will behave. Various scientific disciplines were ranked in a hierarchical taxonomy, based on the extent to which other disciplines were dependent on them for their knowledge base. Positivist philosophy can trace its roots to ancient Greece, and the word 'positive' refers to the notion of the attainment of ultimate truth.

The positivists of the 19th century were the forerunners of the more extreme logical positivists of the 20th century who claimed that legitimate knowledge was conferred solely to that which resulted from hypothetico-deductive methodology. Logical positivism is characterized by the rise of hypothetico-deductivism as the only method of discovering new knowledge. Logical positivists believed that science was about generating assumptions which are based only on observable phenomena. Hypotheses are devised and tested in order to verify a theory or to predict. The phenomena being observed are broken down (reductionism) to smaller parts which are called variables. The hypothetico-deductive methodology introduced by the logical positivists claims to be rational, logical, objective, value-free measurement and is based on truth which can be verified.

The 19th century also saw the origins of a philosophical movement called *existentialism*. The existentialists had a completely new way of explaining knowledge and truth. Kierkegaard (1813–1855), for example, argued that knowledge and truth are subjective. What he suggested was that all really important truths are personal. They are truths which are true for me. Knowledge gained from reason is totally unimportant unless it is important to my existence. We can be absolutely certain of a specific fact – a reasoned truth. But, if it is not fundamental to my existence, it is immaterial. Important knowledge is, therefore, subjective and is only important if it affects my very existence.

Existentialism was also influential in the 20th century and developed blurred boundaries with another philosophical paradigm called *humanism*. Sartre (1905–1980), was a 20th century existentialist who argued that existentialism starts from nothing but humanity itself. Existence, according to Sartre, was more than just being alive. Existence was about being conscious of one's existence. Existence takes priority over all things, including one's nature. Sartre did not believe that human beings have an innate nature. Human beings create themselves. There is no blueprint for life except for the one we each create for our own lives and, because of this, each of us is responsible for everything we do. There are no external norms in existentialism and, as free individuals, we are condemned to make our own choices for which we must take full responsibility. Sartre argued that it is imperative that life has meaning but we must create this meaning in our lives.

Sartre, like many philosophers before him, examined consciousness. But he believed that consciousness does not exist until it has perceived something. Consciousness implies that there is something we are conscious of. Human beings play a part in selecting what we will perceive. At the same time that this existential thinking was taking root in philosophy, the social sciences were developing their own body of knowledge and own world view of knowledge.

Some sociologists and anthropologists conducted their search for knowledge by using the then respected ideas of legitimate knowledge of the positivists. Others like Durkheim (1858–1917), Weber (1864–1920) and Mead (1865–1931), searched for knowledge and truth in ways which reflect alternatives to the hypothetico-deductive approach. Concepts like empathy, reflexivity, personal meaning and lived experience were beginning to emerge as part of legitimate knowledge and method. A new philosophical world view emerged in the 20th century known as *phenomenology* which has its roots in existentialism. Phenomenology acknowledges that reality is personal and, therefore, knowledge is personal. New knowledge comes from seeking to understand an individual's lived experience.

The intention of presenting this selective history of knowledge is several-fold. Firstly, it is to provide an understanding of how the world's understanding and view of knowledge has changed over time. Secondly, it is to demonstrate just how powerfully the history of a positivist, reductionist and rationalist influences our understanding of legitimate knowledge today.

Nursing practice and nursing education has its past and its present in the paradigms of philosophy of knowledge which have been presented. One could argue that the new paradigms of feminism and post-modernism are changing this. These two particular paradigms are examined in Chapter 3.

The third reason for exploring the knowledge paradigms is to examine where, if at all, intuition fits in and where it is and is not addressed within the various paradigms. Gerrity (1987, p. 64) makes the point that scientific enquiry, the 'most rational and logical of our pursuits' could not exist without personal knowing (intuition). Hunches, gut feelings and biases all influence both hypothetical development and scientific method. However, scientists also present their reports and findings in a logical and explicit manner. The hunches and intuitive insights are left out of scientific research reports (Gerrity, 1987, p. 64) which makes it impossible to determine its place in scientific enquiry. It is this that nursing has used as its model for many years. As a result, intuitive and insightful parts of gathering knowledge are largely ignored, undervalued and neglected in nursing.

But in order to examine the place intuition might have in the future of nursing, it seems important to take a clear look at what intuition is.

♦

INTUITION EXPLAINED AND DEFINED

One of the side-effects of nursing's attempt to emerge as a legitimate profession which stands alongside other professional groups has been the need to concern itself with the positivist approach to its knowledge base and rationalistic view of its decision-making processes. In seeking legitimization, nursing has been concerned with developing a scientific platform for its practice and creating a theoretical basis which can be tested by scientific method. Gerrity (1987, p. 63) argues that, as a result of this, the 'scope of enquiry within nursing has become unduly narrowed to processes that are amenable to investigation by direct measurement.'

What is also noticeable is that, as a result of this, both nursing education and our notions of clinical evaluation have followed this pattern. Any nursing experience which does not fit into this positivist, scientific paradigm has been, at best, under-valued and, at worst, ignored.

The emphasis on factual and objective measurement has led to intuition in nursing being under-valued. The new move towards evidence based practice is continuing this trend despite the reality that much of successful and useful nursing has little factual or objective research base except that it works! What is perpetuating in the 1990s was identified by Chenault (1964) over 30 years ago who observed that nursing's 'capitulation to scientism' is based on the assumption that only the 'objective' mind can generate significant professional questions and answers.

Yet recent philosophical enquiry into the nature of knowledge (Hospers, 1990) suggests that legitimate and valuable knowledge comes in at least seven forms: perception, introspection, memory, reason, faith, intuition and testimony. At least three of these are neither testable nor measurable and yet they are recognized as legitimate ways in which human beings come to know something.

If we return to the anecdote related in the beginning, what is clear is that the nurse on the ward began by seeking objective and measurable information, became uncomfortable with its accuracy and was in touch with some intuitive processes inside herself. Perhaps other forms of knowledge identified by Hospers come into play as well. Did she have a memory of previous, similar experiences? Did she perceive something outside that which was defined by the clinical observations (pulse and blood pressure) which she made and recorded? What is clear, however, is that there was no rationality, in the Cartesian sense, behind her decision to ring me. For Descartes, only those things amenable to systematic observation and experiment can be discussed as absolute knowledge in an objective world.

So what does the literature offer in helping to define intuition when the process itself seems inexplicable? Wescott (1968) defines intuition as a process of reaching accurate conclusions based on concensually inadequate information. Clearly, the staff nurse in the story at the beginning of this chapter did just that. Bastik (1982) suggests that intuition is the most perfect form of human thought. Collins English Dictionary (Hanks, 1990, p. 422) defines intuition as 'instinctive knowledge of or belief about something without conscious reasoning.'

Ferguson (1980) calls intuition 'whole, brain knowing' (p. 114) or 'instinctive knowing' (p. 324). Polyani (1966) suggested that we know more than we can say and described this type of intuitive knowledge as tacit knowledge, a concept enlarged upon by Benner and Tanner (1987) who define intuition as understanding without a rationale. Schon's notion of reflection-in-action (see Chapter 6) is based on what he calls knowing-in-action, the intuitive, tacit moment when, in the middle of doing something, we know that it is either right to do it or perhaps wrong and, therefore, we change our course of action (Schon, 1983). What seems to be clear is that intuition is a way in which we come to know something but which bypasses our normal reliance on logic and linear thought processes. It is a way in which we see the whole without controlling the way the whole happens. It is knowledge of a truth, arrived at as a whole, without reliance on the usual conscious reasoning process. There is an ever-growing store of evidence that is showing that, despite our inability to explain it, correct decisions are made in the face of little or no reasoned data.

Jung (1969, p. 441) created the concept of synchronicity, defining it as 'the simultaneous occurrence of a certain psychic state with one or more external events which appear as meaningful parallels to the momentary subjective state, and, in certain cases, vice versa'. He uses the term *synchronicity* to refer to the fact that events occur simultaneously and meaningfully but are not causal to each other. Jung called it a 'coincidence in time' where the two events have a similar meaning or close relationship.

Slater (1992) offers an example of synchronicity, describing a situation where one person has a dream about something or someone, sees/experiences the next day the event or person who was the subject of the dream, and then hears someone else talking about the same subject of the dream. There is no cause involved, it is coincidental, and there is a close relationship in the time of all three events – the dream itself, seeing/experiencing the subject of the dream and hearing someone talk about it. Others have defined synchronicity as a coincidence between a thought or feeling and an external event occurring or when a person has a dream, vision or premonition about something that will happen in the future which then, in fact, happens (Boleni, 1979).

Slater (1992), through the process of concept analysis, demonstrates that intuition is a synchronistic event. She suggests that nurses who are bound by rules and inexperience (novice nurses) are less able to tune into intuitive understanding. Expert nurses, however, learn to trust their intuition and the synchronistic events surrounding them.

Loye (1983) suggests that there are different types of intuition: cognitive inference, Gestalt intuition and precognitive function. What differs across each of the three types is that, within each, a correct decision is arrived at based on fewer and fewer measurable cues, precognitive functions operating with no environmental cues at all and cognitive inference operating in those instances when there are environmental cues (things we see and hear). But they happen so quickly and subliminally that we cannot recall that they influenced the decision we take. What seems to emerge from all of the definitions and ways of explaining intuition is that it has certain characteristics.

Firstly, intuition leads to knowing a fact or truth as a whole; secondly, the getting of this kind of knowledge is immediate (Rew, 1986, p. 23); thirdly, the knowledge we gain is independent of the rationalistic linear process of reasoning, and we are unlikely to be able to explain how we came to know it. It is interesting to consider that science and technology have generated so many options for us but it is only our intuition can help us to choose (Ferguson, 1980).

♦

THE PLACE OF INTUITION IN SCIENCE

Scientific enquiry 'begins as a story about a possible world – a story which we invent and criticise and modify as we go along, so that it ends by being as nearly as we can make it, a story about real life.'

(Medawar, 1969, p. 59)

Medawar (1969) described two caricatures of medical practitioners and how they each might make a clinical diagnosis. The caricature of the first practitioner demonstrates inductive thinking in his approach to making a clinical judgement. The patient comes to the doctor saying that he feels awful and the physician attempts to discover what is wrong. The inductive physician empties himself of all pre-conceived ideas about what might be wrong and observes his patient closely. He records the patient's colour, pulse, respiration and blood pressure; tests his reflexes; tests urine; carries out various blood tests and other investigations as necessary.

When all possible factual evidence is amassed, classified and processed, the inductive practitioner finds a diagnosis which is arrived at by logic and reasoning. Medawar reminds us that this could have all been classified and processed by a computer and the diagnosis would be a right one unless the factual evidence was either incomplete or erroneous. There is no doubt that this is an extreme case and that, in reality, a doctor uses more than facts and evidence. Medawar recognizes that 'flair and insight and the enrichment that long experience brings to clinical skills' (p. 43) is part of the medical diagnostic process.

The problem is, however, that the medical world tends to place higher value on the unbiased observation, the apparatus, the 'ritual of fact finding' (p. 44) and the inductive process which is labelled as scientific. What about the caricature of the second practitioner? He comes to a clinical diagnosis in another way. When the patient enters the doctor's surgery, this second clinician observes his patient with a purpose, with an idea in mind. From the moment the clinician meets the patient, he sets questions for himself, questions which are influenced by some kind of foreknowledge or 'sensory clue' (p. 49). This foreknowledge, sensory clue and set of questions direct his thoughts and guide the clinician towards his new observations which will tell him whether or not his provisional ideas (which are constantly forming) are either acceptable or unsound. This second clinician, according to Medawar, is engaging in 'rapid reciprocation between an imaginative process and a critical process, between imaginative conjecture and critical evaluation (p. 44). As it proceeds, a hypothesis will be formed which provides a reasonable basis for treatment or further tests. Like the first caricature, this second scenario is an archetype, an extreme picture.

What is important about this second, hypothetico-deductive approach is that it suggests that science is not propelled by logic and reasoning. Medawar describes scientific reasoning as:

an exploratory dialogue that can always be resolved into two voices or two episodes of thought,

imaginative and critical, which alternate and interact'
(p. 46).

In the imaginative part of the process we form an opinion,
make an informed guess or have a hunch, and from this we
form a hypothesis. Medawar suggests that this process is
not illogical but rather outside logic. Scientific reasoning
then is a dialogue between the possible and the actual.
There is nothing terribly scientific about the
hypothetico-deductive process. Medawar says that the
process is not even an intellectual one (p. 54). He reminds
us that imagination and inspiration enters into all scientific
reasoning at every level (p. 55). What has emerged in the
western scientific community, however, is a reluctance to
accept that creativity, creative imagination and intuition
are a fundamental component of science and scientific
method. Creativity and imagination are descriptors of
artists not scientists. 'Inventors,' says Medawar (1969, p. 58)
'speak unaffectedly about ... inspirations. Doctors do
not.'
    Intuition appears in many different forms in science
although, regardless of the form, they share commonalities.
The suddenness of their appearances, the wholeness of the
concept they embody and the fact that there is an absence of
conscious thought (Medawar, 1969, p. 56). Medawar
suggests four types of intuition in science:

◆ Deductive intuition – perception or awareness of a
  logical implication suddenly; a raising of awareness.
◆ Inductive intuition – hitting upon a hypothesis which
  will be explained eventually through logic; a creative,
  intuitive and generative act which begins a scientific
  quest.
◆ An instant insight into a real or apparent similarity
  between two or more schemes of ideas. Medawar calls
  this 'wit' (p. 57) although it could be called wisdom, a
  concept which will be discussed later.
◆ Thinking out an experiment, demonstrating creative
  and intuitive flair.

And it was Medawar who, in 1969, pre-dating Schon (1983,
1987) described the process of reflection as a way of
harnessing creativity in the scientific process. Scientific
enquiry is, therefore, a balance between imaginativeness and
critical analysis. Both are necessary to science, and scientific
enquiry cannot exist without both. Neither on its own is

sufficient. Intuition in science makes science more human by contributing to both its successes and its fallibilities.

◆

THE PLACE OF INTUITION IN ART

The reason for including intuition in art in this chapter is to explore the artistry of nursing and the place of intuition in that artistry. In Chapter 1 David Parker explored nursing and art. Much of the literature he cites seems to imply that intuition or tacit knowledge lies within the domain of the artistic (rather than the scientific) side of nursing.

The fundamental difference between art and science seems to lie in the different ways in which decisions are made within the two. Ferguson (1980) suggests that scientific decision-making and knowledge-getting use linear thought patterns. It relies on the left side of the brain which organizes new information into the existing scheme of things (Ferguson, 1980, p. 326). Scientific decision-making relies on calculations and measurement, artistic decision-making comes from sensing and intuiting and tacit knowledge (Polanyi, 1967) which we can neither measure nor explain. Art, creation, insight and intuition are not linear processes. These are mediated in the right half of the brain which cannot verbalize what it knows (Ferguson, 1980, p. 326). The right half of the brain produces symbols, images and metaphors (all components of art) which need to be both recognized and reformulated in the left hemisphere of the brain in order for that information to be wholly known. The right half of the brain sees the context in which information exists and, therefore, it also provides meaning.

Ferguson suggests (p. 326) that every forward leap in progress throughout history has been the result of right-brain insights seeing the whole, perceiving relationships and processing novelty. Bastick (1982), in his theory of intuition, describes it as a universal ability which is reflected in the creative inspirations of scientists as well as in the hunches of daily life which guide individual behaviour. What is important in this definition of intuition is, firstly, in the phrase 'creative inspirations.' This is the language of art. One dictionary definition of art is 'human creativity as distinguished from nature' (Hanks, 1990). Intuition as creative intuition places it firmly within art. Secondly, Bastick singles out scientists as the users of this creative inspiration, thus using intuition to bridge the gap between art and science.

Scientific decision-making uses linear processes to reach conclusions or generate knowledge. Decision-making in art, however, is an 'unstructured mode of reasoning' (Kahneman and Tversky, 1982) which relies on processes other than reasoning to reach conclusions.

Ellis (1982) explored the concept of discovery and suggested that discovery is individual to the person doing the discovering. 'It can be serendipitous' (p. XI) and is a function of such things as interest, opportunity, personality, chance and creativity.

Again, Ellis uses the language of art to explain the intuitive process. Art is subjective and personal. A person's response to art will be unique to that person. Earlier in this chapter there is reference to Locke's notion of primary and secondary quality. Secondary qualities are sensations like colour, smell, taste and sound. They are not the real qualities within that which is creating the sensation (a painting, a cordon bleu dinner, a symphony). Rather, they reproduce the effect of the painting, the cordon bleu dinner or the symphony on our senses.

All art produces secondary qualities of sensation, individual to the person doing the sensing. I can know that a piece of music is beautiful because it is beautiful to me. I cannot use words to make it beautiful for you. Schraeder and Fischer (1986) make the point that nursing is artful expression which takes place on an intuitive level. I know when the art of nursing is beautiful because it is beautiful to me. I may try my best to explain the beauty of a nursing action to you but I cannot use words to make it beautiful for you. I know intuitively that it is so.

Art also relies on imagination which is defined in the Collins English Dictionary (Hanks, 1990, p. 415). as 'mental creative ability'. Mental creative ability is what the artist demonstrates as the starting point and the driver for the art. Doering (1992) suggests that both experience and imagination (creative ability) contribute to intuition.

Intuition has a place in science as well as a place in art. Too often in our dualistic world we see art and science in conflict with each other. However, Benner and Tanner (1987) remind us that ' intuitive knowledge and analytic reasoning are not in an either/or opposition; they can – and often do – work together.' In synchronicity, meaningful coincidence that has no discernible cause (Jung, 1969),

Slater concludes that the expert nurse is one who appreciates the synchronistic events around us and can blend together intuitive knowledge and analytic reasoning.

◆

WISDOM IN NURSING: INTUITION, JUDGEMENT AND CLINICAL DECISION-MAKING

Wisdom is the ability to use one's experience and knowledge to make sensible decisions or judgements. One of the factors which may be preventing nursing fully developing its wisdom, is the over-concern with having a scientific base for its practice and with developing a theory that can be tested using scientific methods (Gerrity, 1987). Wisdom relies on an expanded scope of enquiry, knowledge and experience. The concern with science and scientific method has narrowed nursing into processes that are amenable to directly measurable investigation (Gerrity, 1987). Scientific knowledge is not sufficient for nursing to cultivate its wisdom.

In recent years there has been a value shift in our understanding of nursing knowledge and experience with many writers (Benner, 1984; Pyles and Stern, 1983; Schraeder and Fischer, 1986) recognizing both the need for intuitive knowledge to be accepted as legitimate nursing knowledge and the accuracy of intuitive judgement. Wisdom in clinical decision-making relies on practice which reflects all types of knowledge and all types of decision-making. Gerrity (1987) reminds us that changing paradigms in the nature of scientific inquiry came about with the realization that linear, verbal and intellectual knowing is not the only way available (Ornstein, 1972). Even scientific inquiry needed other forms of knowledge to move forward.

Carl Jung contributed to changing the way we understand the role of sensing and intuition in judgement (Jung, 1933). Jung's theory proposes that all conscious mental activity can be classified into four mental processes. Two of these – sensing and intuition – are perceptive processes, and the other two – thinking and feeling – are judgement processes. At any one time, things enter our consciousness either through our senses or our intuition. That which we are continually sensing or intuiting (if we remain in a conscious state) is sorted, classified, analysed and evaluated by the two judgement processes of thinking and feeling.

Sensing establishes what exists (Gerrity, 1987) and makes

us aware of what is happening at the present moment. Intuition is a perception of what is possible, of meanings and of relationships, all as a result of insight. It is a hunch, a creative discovery, and enables that which is beyond the visible, beyond the present, to be perceived.

Thinking is the mental process of judgement that helps us make logical connections. It consists of analytical processes, problem solving and objectivity. Feeling, the second of the two judgement processes, is the mental activity through which we reach decisions by weighing up relative values and merits related to issues and experiences. As such, it is a more subjective type of judgement process. When we use these processes to make judgements, we are more likely to be aware of the values of others as well as those of our own. (Gerrity, 1987)

Jung suggested that, although everyone who is in a state of consciousness uses all four mental processes (Jung, 1933), each individual will have an innate preference for one (or more) over the others. Gerrity (1987) suggests that nurses tend to have preference for sensing as a perceptual process and have lesser developed intuitive processes. Myers and Myers (1980) suggest that, when lesser developed processes are not used, they become 'imprisoned processes of the mind ... if they are suppressed ... they eventually break out and come up to consciousness' (p. 202).

Myers and Myers (1980), Gerrity (1987) and others all believe that lesser developed processes can become more developed in tandem with the need to further develop those processes for which they show preference. Each of the perceptual processes has a place. Sensing allows us to be aware and attuned to what is happening now and the relevant information or facts. Intuition allows nurses to know what changes are taking place in the absence of measurable signs. This also requires an awareness of the relevant facts. Benner (1984) states quite clearly that expert nurses do not rely overly on their intuitive processes but, at the same time, they trust their intuitive processes and do not ignore them. Wisdom in nursing then suggests that clinical judgements are based both on what we sense and on our intuition.

Problem-solving care plans (the nursing process) rely primarily on sensory information. The potential for harnessing the intuitive is limited in this linear form of decision-making. Care plans, according to Gerrity (1987), are not used because they are self-limiting and do not represent the intuitive knowledge which underpins much of effective, appropriate, caring intuitive judgements.

Where care plans do seem to be used, it is likely that this is due to those nurses disregarding much intuitive data that is a part of expert nursing. Care plans divide the patient into parts (called problems or potential problems) which need to be solved or prevented. In doing this, the patient is seen in parts, and the whole, which is the basis of intuition, is lost. Expert nursing is then lost and wisdom in nursing cannot emerge; they become a hidden face of the cube.

Benner's main argument (1984) is that skill acquisition from novice to expert is about changes in perceptual ability from stage to stage. The expert nurse experiences a Gestalt (an organized whole picture) of a situation, has hunches or 'ah ha' experiences which are treated as serious information and are followed up with a search for evidence to confirm that hunch (Benner, 1984). Through this intuitive process, the expert nurse views the patient in terms of what is possible. Expert nurses do not use the nursing process or nursing models for making clinical judgements (Field, 1987).

Nursing wisdom then would be described as the coming together of well-developed sensing and intuition processes with equally well-developed feeling and thinking processes to make expert clinical judgements. This is not about forming a more complete science of nursing, as suggested by Gerrity (1987, p. 70). Rather, it is a way of creating a wisdom of nursing which marries artistry with science into something which is greater than both.

Conversation

CHAPTER 6	*Through what you've said, I've really come to appreciate that intuition is as important as other forms of knowledge. Nurses seem to use intuition in their day to day work, without being aware of it, or indeed valuing it.*
CHAPTER 5	*Yes, but remember that this is an historical problem about the legitimacy of types of knowledge. What I did was to show that some very good nursing decisions can be made in ways that nurses cannot explain rationally. We call this intuition.*
CHAPTER 6	*You also ended with a discussion about wisdom. One of the ways nurses become wise is through knowing these decisions and valuing them.*
CHAPTER 5	*It's not just decisions that have been made, it is also about ideas nurses have yet to try out.*
CHAPTER 6	*I agree. I'm going to talk about experimenting with, and caring for, ideas, through reflection....*

THINKING AND CARING: NEW PERSPECTIVES ON REFLECTION

Diane Marks-Maran and Pat Rose

There is a growing body of literature related to reflection on, and reflection in, practice. In this chapter we will review this literature, and examine it in relation to ways of knowing. We will explore a use for reflection, that is reflection in caring for an idea, which has received less attention in the literature, and discuss the use of Socratic dialogue as a reflection tool. Finally we will demonstrate some of the ideas using examples from our own experience.

Nursing education and teacher education has increasingly been influenced by the work of Argyris and Schon (1974) and by Schon (1983, 1987). Our understanding of reflection in and on practice is based on a fundamental assumption put forward by Langford (1973), who suggested that all human action is undertaken to achieve a purpose or to execute an intention. This implies that all human actions, including nursing action, reflects ideas, models or some kind of theoretical notion of purposes and intentions and how these purposes and intentions can be executed. These theoretical notions could be called 'theories of action' or 'action theories'. Argyris and Schon (1974) observed that many people say one thing (theory) and do something completely different (action), embodied on the phrase 'He does not practice what he preaches'. This observation led Argyris and Schon to suggest two types of action theories: *espoused theories* (our stated purpose or intention) and *theories-in-use* (our attempt to put our stated intention or purpose into action). Espoused theories then, are those theories which practitioners claim to believe in, and deliberately set out to communicate to others. Theories-in-use are the theories which influence or govern what we actually do in practice. The large body of literature about a 'theory–practice gap' suggests that there is evidence that the espoused theories (those consciously learned from teachers and from the literature) held by nurses do not match up with theories-in-use (that which actually happens in clinical practice). Theories-in-use tend to be learned informally, and usually unconsciously, by nurses through repetition in day to day experience. As such, theories-in-use may be very different from espoused theories.

Greenwood (1993) cites a number of research studies of nursing practice (theories-in-use) where the findings demonstrate that nurses focus their care on diseases, not on the whole person; that nursing care is about getting through the work at all cost and through adhering to routine; and that the technical work is 'real' nursing while day-to-day activities are 'just basic care' (Kelly, 1991; Seed, 1991, French, 1992). A key observation made by Greenwood (1993) is that, in principle, espoused theories and theories-in-use can be identical. Alternatively, they may be different yet be compatible with each other. They can, however, be different and also be incompatible. Practitioners can be unaware of the incompatibility between their espoused theories and their theories-in-use.

The increasing importance now being placed upon evidence-based practice suggests that there is a growing demand for nurses to maintain a closer compatibility between their espoused theories (research evidence) and their theories-in-action (actual nursing care). Current practice, however, suggests that when there are incompatibilities between espoused theories and theories-in-use, it is the latter which tends to govern what happens in the messy world of nursing. Because of this, it is important to identify and explicate existing theories-in-use in nursing and, on an individual level, to have the opportunity to understand our own theories-in-use, to learn about our own effectiveness as nurses, to compare our theories-in-use with our espoused theories and perhaps to make new decisions about the way we work.

Greenwood (1993) goes on to discuss the contribution of Sloboda who made the point that the function of real work situations is to give meaning to subsequent experiences of similar situations and to make then more manageable. Human beings construct theories-in-use through repeated experience of similar or the same experiences. These theories-in-use are then triggered when a similar situation or experience arises again.

In nursing, according to Greenwood (1993), our espoused theories are triggered by situations where we are expected to demonstrate these espoused theories, such as in presenting assignments for nursing courses we undertake, and in teaching nursing, both in the classroom, and in the clinical area. They are also triggered by those assessing the suitability for nursing students of that clinical area. In contrast to espoused theories, theories-in-use, are triggered by totally different stimuli, including the patients' situation, interactions with their relatives, and doctors or other colleagues. The question is: how do we create theories-in-use through our experiences?

♦

FINDING MEANING IN THEORIES-IN-USE

Schon (1983, 1987) suggested the term 'technical rationality' to describe a pure applied science view of any professional practice. Technical rationality is a product of the positivist philosophical paradigm which emerged in the early part of the 20th century as a way of explaining the scientific and technical triumphs of the time. In many respects, the advent of positivism owes its roots to a long history since the 1700s when science, technology and industry began to shape our society. The scientific paradigm, or world view, is a powerful and dominant one which led to the general assumption that human progress is achieved by using science to advance technology which then leads to achievement of human purpose. Technical rationality, as a by-product of this positivist philosophy, is based on the assumption that problem-solving, using scientific theory, method and technique, will lead to rigorous professional practice.

It is this same positivist philosophy that underpins both the concept of nursing process and the concept of evidence-based practice. Schon (1983) also suggested that systematic problem-solving presupposes one or both of two things: firstly, that problems are already defined or easily definable, and/or secondly, that the goals or solutions are clear fixed and universally agreed. Recent approaches to nursing also seem to assume that nursing decisions are made in this systematic, problem-solving, tidy, positivistic way. The reality for nurses, however, is that problems in practice are not tidy; they are not easy to label. Real-life nursing problems are 'messy' and contain any number of uncertainties, instability, uniqueness and value conflict (Greenwood, 1993).

Problem-understanding and problem-solving, however, cannot be achieved by science alone. Identifying a problem relies on a nurse's ability to make sense of a situation and find meaning within it. In practice, this happens through theories-in-use which have been created from repeated exposure to similar situations. Schon (1983, 1987) and Greenwood (1993) suggest that, in any given clinical situation, the nurse selects which aspect to attend to. In doing so, the nurse uses (consciously or unconsciously) interpretative frameworks, rather than linear problem-solving processes, to structure the situation. Schon refers to this as 'interactive naming and framing' and says that it reflects the professional activity of practice. This interactive naming and framing process is non-technical and it enables the nurse to clarify the ends and means within the situation. Each situation will have its own interpretation and meaning. Technical rationality and systematic problem-solving just does not work in the real world of work. We would suggest that the problem-solving or nursing process approach to nursing is, in fact, a way of nurses recording events *after* they have taken place (reflection-after-action) using a framework which does not actually reflect how nursing decisions were made.

♦

REFLECTION AS THE COUNTER-BALANCE TO TECHNICAL RATIONALITY

Schon suggests that the limitations of technical rationality can be overcome by creating an epistemology of practice where technical problem solving exists within a broader framework of reflective enquiry or reflective practice. Schon (1987) suggests that there are two constituent elements of reflective practice: reflection-in-action and reflection-on-action. Schon describes reflection-in-action as thinking about what you are doing while you are doing it. Reflection-in-action is characterized by something which surprises or puzzles practitioners, while they are in the process of undertaking a professional activity, and results in a practitioner asking (consciously or subconsciously) key questions in the midst of the action. These questions might be:

- ◆ What am I noticing here and what does it mean?
- ◆ What judgements am I making and by what criteria?
- ◆ What am I doing and why?
- ◆ Is there an alternative course of action other than the one I am taking?

Through these questions, the nurse is reflecting on the understandings which have been implicit in the activities, the feeling which led to the original decision to take a certain action, and the way the initial problem was structured. These things, which were once unconscious, now come to the surface, are critically examined, restructured and results in a different course of action being taken than the one which the nurses started out to do. In summary, reflection-in-action enables the nurse to reshape action while that action is taking place. It is a spiral thought process, leading to change in practice, and this is what is different from the linear process of a systematic, positivist, problem-solving model. It is how it is in the real but messy world of nursing.

Reflection-on-action is described by Greenwood (1993) as a 'cognitive post-mortem'. It involves looking back on a past experience, exploring again the understandings that were present at the time of the experience and creating new understandings in light of the outcomes of the original action.

Both reflection-in-action and reflection-on-action are ways of identifying, testing and changing someone's theories-in-use. Reflection, then, is a way in which professionals create new understandings of knowledge in practice.

◆

TYPES OF KNOWLEDGE AND WAYS OF KNOWING

Many writers, including Carper (1978), Schon (1983, 1987), Polanyi (1958), Habermas (1972), and Hospers (1990), have offered taxonomies for identifying types of knowledge. The following discussion illustrates that there are certain similarities and some differences across these different taxonomies.

Scientific knowledge

Carper (1978) described empirical or scientific knowledge as 'knowledge that is systematically organised into general laws and theories for the purpose of describing, explaining and predicting phenomena of special concern to the discipline of nursing'. Argyris and Schon (1974) refer to this as espoused theory as described above, and suggest it fits in the same category as empirical or scientific theory. It was this view which led Schon (1983, 1987), in his later works, to describe scientific knowledge as technical rationality, to indicate a pure applied science point of view of professional practice.

That nursing has its early 20th century history rooted in the medical model is a direct result of the rise of positivism, and the scientific paradigm in the 1930s. The value placed on scientific knowledge as the important knowledge underpinning nursing has led to nursing's emphasis on research-based practice in the 1970s and 1980s, hard facts and objectively (Reed and Proctor, 1993), and more recently, the move within all of health care towards evidence-based practice.

In Schon's definition of technical rationality, scientific knowledge is generated by academics and transmitted to students who are then expected to put it into action (Schon, 1983). Two assumptions underpin this: first, that research and evidence is a superior form of knowledge, and secondly that there is always evidence to support practice decisions. Miller (1985) and Greenwood (1984) both argue that the flaw in this assumption is that in reality, science tends to produce irrelevant abstractions which cannot really inform practice. Scientific method also assumes that knowledge is more important than the subjects (people) it serves.

Practical knowledge

Practical knowledge is that which is gained from the experience of professional practice. Whereas scientific knowledge comes from a hypothetico-deductive, positivist paradigm, practical knowledge is inductive, and uses reflection to identify and articulate the knowledge gained from practice.

It is important to differentiate practical knowledge from ritual, habit, or custom and practice. The latter is practice without reflection, the former is practice with knowledge arising from reflecting on that practice. Ritual and habit in professional practice have been described extensively in the literature (Walsh and Ford, 1989; Mezirow, 1988). There is a relationship between practical knowledge and theories-in-use (Argyris and Schon, 1974) in that theories-in-use are those theories which nurses learn through their everyday practice (Greenwood, 1993) rather than through books, or lectures or formal learning. However, theories-in-use without reflection can actually help nurses to remain oblivious to their own effectiveness or ineffectiveness (Argyris and Schon, 1974). Schon (1987) argued that in order to move away from only relying on technical rationality, or ineffective theories-in-use, the professional needs to build up practical knowledge through reflection-on-action and reflection-in-action.

Practical knowledge is knowledge gained from practice. It is not the same as just perpetuating custom and practice. Friedson (1971) claimed that in a professional culture, the practitioners seem to be self-validating and self-confirming. They have no time to debate or discuss the uncertainties of their practice. They must believe that what they are doing is right at the time. Eraut (1985) confirms that in saying that in times of 'hot action' there is no time for discussion or debate because of the immediacy of the situation. Professionals find evaluation of their actions difficult and painful because it takes too much time, is stressful, risky and de-skilling (Friedson, 1971). Eraut (1985) argues for a time set aside for professional to escape from the practice setting, and to reflect on that practice away from the 'hot action'.

To summarize, practical knowledge is knowledge gained from the process of debating, discussing and reflecting on real practice situation. Without reflection, practical knowledge cannot develop and expand.

Personal knowledge: intuition and tacit knowledge

Carper (1978) described personal knowledge of self as one of the four domains of nursing knowledge. Personal knowledge is about an individual's experience of becoming self-aware. As Carper (1978) stated: 'One does not know about the self, one strives simply to know the self.' Carper argues that it is only through being self-aware and knowing oneself that one can know and understand others. We do not communicate personal knowledge through language. Rather, we communicate our personal knowledge through our existence; through who we are. The process of reflection enables us as human beings to know ourselves, and use ourselves as healers. Rew and Barrow (1987) suggest that this is the intuition part of nursing, the art of nursing, which provides the personal knowledge which underpins many nursing decisions and action.

Polyani (1967) suggests that 'we know more than we can say'. This is what tacit knowledge is. It is complementary to Benner and Tanner (1987) who describe intuition as 'understanding without a rationale'. Schon (1987) describes tacit knowledge as a key component of reflection-in-action. He uses the term 'knowing-in-action' to describe that intuitive moment when we know as we are doing something that is right to do at that very second, even when we cannot explain why we know it. That intuitive, tacit moment can also be that time when we know, despite all the evidence, that it is wrong to take a certain action.

Benner (1984) suggests that central to good nursing judgement is perceptual awareness, and that this begins with vague hunches and assessments which seem to by-pass critical analysis. She found that expert nurses frequently describe their judgements and decisions as being a result of gut feelings, or a feeling that something isn't quite right. An example of this appears at the beginning of Chapter 5.

Hospers (1990) reveals great variety in the way human beings come to 'know' something, listing seven ways of knowing: perception, introspection, memory, reason, faith, intuition, and testimony. Evidential or scientific knowledge, therefore, may arise from reason. Tacit knowledge, however, arises from intuition, perception and even faith. Hospers strongly argues that there is no order of importance in these seven ways of knowing. If we accept that personal knowledge is as valid as scientific knowledge then we should therefore be more confident in using it as justification for our actions.

Schon (1983) was describing tacit, intuitive knowledge when he said: 'When we go about the spontaneous intuitive performance of our actions of everyday life, we show ourselves to be knowledgeable in a special way'. He went on to acknowledge that, when we try to describe intuitive knowledge, we often find ourselves lost for words, or we produce descriptions which are inappropriate. He said: 'Our knowing is ordinarily tacit....It seems right to say our knowing is our action'.

In summary, nursing is not merely empirical knowledge arising from reason, evidence and problem solving, and yet it is partially about these things. Nursing is also not merely intuition, yet it is also partially about these things. Neither is nursing the sum of the two sets of things, the sum of art and science. We would suggest that nursing is more than the sum of art and science, just as a cube is more than the sum of its faces, and that to try to describe the whole of nursing as the sum of these arbitrary parts does little to explain either the knowledge base of nursing or the practice of nursing.

Nursing is more than, and greater than, the sum of art and science, and at times it is neither art nor science, but it is always nursing. Nursing's uniqueness lies not in trying to define its parts nor in arguing for nursing as an art and/or science. Instead, understanding the uniqueness of nursing comes from developing reflection in and on action as a normal skill and activity within our practice. In doing so, we will begin to use all forms of knowledge to underpin our practice and create a way of practising which is more than art and science; a way of practising which is nursing.

♦

THE NATURE AND PURPOSE OF REFLECTION

Reflection then, is for finding meaning in theories-in-use, and for developing the various ways of knowing in nursing. It is a journey of experience and an experience of journey. Johns (1992) defines reflective practice as follows: 'Reflection is a reflexive method of gaining access to an understanding of experience which enable practitioners to develop increasing effectiveness of personal action within the conflict of their work'. He continues by offering the suggestion that reflection enables practitioners to bridge the gap between espoused theories (what we say we ought to do) and theories on action (what we really do), saying: 'Reflection involves a commitment to personal confrontation to expose the contradictions between what the practitioner aims to achieve and the way they practice. It is the conflict caused by these contradictions that empowers the practitioner to take necessary actions'.

Effective action is the application of professional judgement which is developed through a reflective cycle, where knowledge is uncovered, assimilated, applied to practice and reflected upon (Johns, 1992). The nature of reflection is such that there is a need for commitment on the part of the practitioner, the need to focus on the nature of the action and what constitutes effectiveness in that action and the realization that professional judgement is the hallmark of professional practice. Reflection is an activity to develop personal, practical or intuitive knowledge. Johns (1992) in referring to Carper's four domains of nursing knowledge, suggests that three of Carper's domains – ethical knowledge, aesthetic knowledge and personal knowledge – can only be learned by reflection and that it is only through reflection that the fourth of Carper's knowledge domains, empirical knowledge (scientific knowledge) can be assimilated effectively into practice. This suggests a first purpose for reflection is to re-define our understanding of nursing knowledge and how nursing knowledge is learned.

A second purpose of reflection is for the development of personal knowledge, or self-awareness. Self-awareness is the development of new personal understandings and insights. It is characterized by new perspectives (seeing an old situation in a new light), changes in behaviour, readiness or application of new knowledge and a commitment to action. Boud et al (1985) offer a reflective learning cycle, the outcome of which is characterized by just these things.

Much of the literature on reflection highlights the skills required to reflect on experience. Self-awareness skills are often identified as necessary for this process (Burnard, 1991; Atkins and Murphy, 1993). Boud et al (1985) appear to be suggesting that the process of reflection *develops* self-awareness; Atkins and Murphy (1993) on the other hand, seem to be suggesting that self-awareness skills are needed in order to engage in reflection. Johns' (1993) model for structured supervised reflection appears to reconcile the two, demonstrating that some self-awareness is required to both identify that there is a need for reflection and to start the process of reflection going.

A third purpose of reflection is to evaluate the appropriateness of our actions, and in discussing this, it is helpful to re-examine the different types of reflection. As noted earlier, Schon (1983) describes two types of reflection, reflection-in-action and reflection-on-action. It seems however that some confusion has arisen over the distinction between the two, and perhaps there are in truth three types of reflection.

Reflection-before-action has not been discussed by Schon. Reed and Proctor (1993) however, discuss this type of reflection in depth. Reflection before action involves thinking through a situation or scenario prior to taking action. It involves critical thinking skills and critical analysis skills (Birx, 1993; Jones and Brown, 1993). Reflection before action enables nurses to use technical rationality, scientific knowledge, empirical knowledge and evidence.

Reed and Proctor (1993) argue that in reflecting before action, practitioners modify and select theories, in creative ways, to fit immediate practice problems. We suggest that this enables evidence to influence practice decisions when such evidence exists. The practitioner reflects on the reality of the situation, and selects judiciously from the espoused theories already learned. Reflecting before action brings knowledge and action together through selecting and rejecting scientific or empirical knowledge and evidence to plan in advance how to solve or manage a real-life situation.

Reflection-during-action describes Schon's reflection-in-action (1983). Sometimes, as we put into action a decision we made (possibly as a result of reflecting-before-action), something takes us by surprise, or puzzles us, or we notice and observe something unexpected. In trying to make sense of this new awareness, we start asking ourselves some questions. We, in effect, stop, even for a few seconds, in the middle of an action. This is reflection-during-action, or 'stopping during'. Reflection-during-action brings our puzzlement or 'aha' to the surface, analysing the thing or things we've noticed, or become aware of, and begins to restructure, reconstruct, or even question our theories, ideas, knowledge or beliefs. It may lead to a change to our planned course of action. These changes, however, may be evidence-based or they may not. They may be intuitive. Often, they will be tacit – we will be certain that something is right or wrong without being able to explain why, and we change our course of action in the middle of that action.

Reflection-after-the-action is the third type of reflection and corresponds to Schon's (1983) reflection-on-action or Greenwood's (1993) cognitive post mortem. Reflecting-after-the-action is when a practitioner, in a structured way, looks back on an experience, explores the knowledge and understanding she brought to the experience, explores the experience of the situation and new knowledge and understanding gained from the experience. We would suggest that the difference between knowledge and understanding one brings to a new situation and the knowledge and understanding one takes away from a new situation is called *learning*. It is through the process of reflection that this difference is identified.

To return to the third purpose of reflection, to evaluate the appropriateness of one's actions, it seems clear that this purpose of reflection employs reflection-after-the-action. The framework for structured reflection offered by Johns (1993) is a framework for reflecting-after-the action to both evaluate the effectiveness of care as well as to become aware of practical knowledge gained from the experience. This leads to a fourth purpose of reflection, to change nursing practice. Again, Johns (1993) equates structured reflection with changing practice. Others, however, warn against expecting reflection to change practice. 'At present, this body of (practical) knowledge is an extremely delicate plant, and to burden it with the responsibility for changing existing views of practice and knowledge is to ask the impossible' (Reed and Proctor, 1993, p. 27). Reed and Proctor (1993) also warn that practice knowledge generated through reflection could become a vehicle by which nursing exchanges one set of rituals for another. This links with a final suggested purpose of reflecting on practice which is to test ritual, habit or custom and practice (Docking, 1993). Testing ritualized nursing can be carried out through reflection before, during and after action.

In summary, the process of reflection enables both personal and practical knowledge to be generated and enables learning to take place. The process of reflection also exposes and resolves contradictions between espoused theories (what we say is good practice) and theories-in-use (what we do).

What has been discussed so far is the way in which reflection can be used in relation to practice. However reflection has wider application in the generation of nursing knowledge. Whilst the importance of sound scientific research in nursing cannot be over-emphasized, it is recognized that there are some questions which science cannot answer (Kikuchi and Simmons, 1992), and that there is therefore also a need for philosophical or 'blue skies' thinking, and this has been incorporated into the strategy for research in nursing in the UK (RCN and RCM, 1993). Such thinking requires a creative approach, in which new ideas are grappled with in the search for solutions to difficult problems and disharmonies, and the answers to gaps in knowledge (Torrence, 1964). May (1994) suggests that scientific knowledge is changing such that previously held universal 'facts', for example in the field of quantum physics and the nature and origin of matter, are now being blown apart as new realities emerge. She argues therefore that creative and intuitive thinking are essential if the findings of science are to be reassessed and explored anew. She adds that this is not only the case in the field of hard sciences but also in social and health sciences.

Munhall (1993) contributes to these ideas by suggesting a cyclical continuum in the search for knowledge in which a new phenomenon is described, theory proposed and hypothesis tested. This results in validation of the theory, but as it is re-evaluated over time, she argues that exceptions to the rule are identified which lead to the possibility of new, but closely related phenomena which need to be described. Thus the cycle of investigation and discovery continues. We would contend that one of the roles of the creative thinker is to seek out the nuances in accepted theory, rather than wait until they appear accidentally. This is an important feature in post-positivist thinking, in which it is acknowledged that all inquiry, far from being objective, is value-bound. For example, researchers introduce their values by the subjects they choose to study, the methodology and methods by which they collect and analyse data and the context in which the work is undertaken (Boyd, 1993). As long as knowledge gained in this value laden way is accepted as fact it will lead to a distorted view of the world. If however, we acknowledge that all knowledge, rather than being truth, is an expression of human interpretation (Munhall, 1993), there will be room for creative thinking and the articulation of new ideas.

This way of thinking is particularly important in nursing in an era in which the delivery of individualized care is not only a key concept but is required of nurses. Our professional body, the UKCC (1992a), states that nurses must 'recognise and respect the uniqueness and dignity of each patient and client....' (clause 7). In order to do this nurses have to acknowledge that every human individual is indeed unique, and that no two will need exactly the same nursing care. Nurses must therefore work within a philosophy which accepts that whilst some aspects of practice can be based on objective science, ultimately our care must be subjective, and the nuances of nursing theory and practice must reflect the differences of the individuals for whom we care.

◆

REFLECTION IN CARING FOR AN IDEA

Mayeroff (1971, p. 11) says: 'In working out a philosophical concept the need to reflect on it again and again from similar and dissimilar points of view is not a burden forced on me; I am simply caring for the idea.' In his philosophy of the nature of caring, he suggests that caring involves helping another to grow and actualize, and that whether the caring is that of husband for wife, parent for child, teacher for pupil, or psychotherapist for patient, the caring will result in a 'qualitative transformation of the relationship'. He goes on to suggest that the same can be true in caring for 'a philosophical or an artistic idea'. He suggests that whether the caring is for a person or an idea there is a common pattern of helping the other grow. In doing this the carer will not impose a direction of growth on the cared for, but will be guided by its own direction.

As part of caring Mayeroff (1971) suggests there must be devotion to that which is cared for, but because of the dependence on the carer for growth, the devotion carries with it obligations. However, the carer does not experience the obligations as burdensome. 'The father who goes for the doctor in the middle of the night for his sick child does not experience this as a burden; he is simply caring for the child' says Mayeroff (1971, p. 11). In the same way the thinker who reflects again and again on an idea does not experience this as a burden, simply as 'caring for the idea', and this caring will result in a qualitative transformation of the idea as it grows. Thus another purpose for reflection in nursing is in caring for ideas.

A number of writers (Schon, 1983, 1987; Boud et al, 1985; Johns, 1993; Reed and Procter, 1993) offer models for engaging in reflection, many of which are presented as a cycle. All these models offer different approaches to what is essentially a process involving awareness, decision, doing, noticing, doing differently, finding meaning, new awareness, learning. These things happen in a different order depending on whether someone is reflecting before action, during action or after the action. Nevertheless, they all are part of the process. Whatever the model of reflection used, it is there to enable these activities to take place, regardless of the order in which they happen. These models for application of reflection to practice, are, however, largely designed to facilitate reflection after the action.

Having discussed nature and purposes of reflection, and introduced the role of reflection in the creative thinking processes using Mayeroff's (1971) concept of caring for an idea, our purpose now is to explore this further using a reflection cycle in demonstrating the role of reflection. It is important to remember that it is not the idea itself, but the process of caring for it, which is the focus. The origins of the idea will be discussed and the personal growth necessary to embark on caring for the idea will be examined. Finally, the idea itself will be explored. As the discussion represents the real experience of an individual, first person descriptions will be given as appropriate (Webb, 1992b).

The idea

I have been a nurse for 25 years, and will always be glad I made nursing my chosen profession. As my career has progressed, like many, I have been disillusioned at times. However, I have never doubted the value of nurses or nursing in the care of the sick and support of the well. Like many others also, I have been aware of an element of my role which I have never been able to fully articulate, and until recently and never seen any attempt by others to articulate. Nevertheless I have always felt compelled to give every ounce of my energy into fulfilling that elusive something within nursing.

The work of two eminent nurses has moved me some way towards understanding what it is I am doing when I am nursing. Jocelyn Lawler (1991) has described the way in which nurses give, sometimes intimate, care to patients in a way in which both patient and nurse feel comfortable, for example, staying with someone who is sitting on a toilet, or cleaning up someone who has been incontinent, in a dignified way. Pam Smith (1992) describes the effort needed to undertake activities such as this successfully as the emotional labour of nursing. Emotional labour in nursing, could be described as work done, for wages, to induce or suppress feeling in order to portray an outward appearance that produces in patients the sense of being cared for in a safe environment. For me, it is that which is created by this emotional labour which draws me to nursing, but what is it?

One day I was sitting in the middle of a ward, waiting for handover to finish so I could talk to a student. As I waited I watched the care given to a child returning from theatre. He was seven years old and had had a fractured arm reduced under general anaesthetic. As he was transferred from the trolley to the bed it was clear that he was only half awake. He was sobbing and crying loudly for his mother who was not present. The nurse leaned right over him, cradled his head against her shoulder with one arm, and rocked him while she quietly soothed him and reassured him that his mother would return soon. In her other hand she held the fingers of his injured arm. As she calmed him she gently suggested that he hold her hand and squeeze it if he was scared. By her creative actions the nurse not only calmed her patient, but also checked the circulation to the fingers of the injured limb by feeling the warmth and movement of his fingers. Shortly, this nurse was called to hand over her patients and another nurse went to the, now quiet, little boy. Without speaking she lifted back the bedcovers and lifted his injured arm. He began to sob and cry for his mother again. The nurse spoke to him loudly, over his cries, telling him to wiggle his fingers. He responded by crying even louder and pulling his arm away from her.

I was very aware of the different approaches of the two nurses and pondered on the meaning of the incident for many weeks. I felt that what the first nurse did was an example of the art of nursing. But this was not enough. What I had seen was art in itself, something beautiful to look at in the same way that music, dancing, poetry or painting are beautiful. The second nurse, on the other hand had created disorder and it was not beautiful to see. For the first time I was struck by the idea that nursing may be an art form in itself, just like painting or poetry. This was the beginning of the idea I will use here to illustrate the concept of reflection in caring for an idea. I had no notion of where this thinking would lead me, but for some months I held onto this seed of an idea, much as the seed of a plant is held in the winter earth waiting for the warmth of spring to transform it. The spring came for my idea when I took the opportunity to explore the nature of nursing as an art. I began by examining the literature on nursing and art.

Carper (1978) describes aesthetics: the art of nursing as one of four patterns of knowing in nursing. She describes aesthetic knowing as expressive and made visible through action to the patient involved who is transformed by it. Carper does not however suggest that aesthetic knowing in nursing equates with theory of aesthetics in art, that is, the notion of beauty and the emotions thus evoked (Sheppard, 1987). Instead she links it with empathy, 'the capacity for participating in or vicariously experiencing another's feelings'. She does however suggest that, through aesthetic knowing, the design of nursing care will have a sense of form and unity in the way in which it is structured.

Watson (1981) in her discourse on 'Nursing's scientific quest' made reference to art forms by suggesting that the motivation of both art and science is the same. She states that 'science is nothing else than the search to discover unity in the wild variety of nature or...in the variety of our experiences. Poetry, painting, the arts are the same search...'. Thus she argued that discoveries in science are a creation in the same way as original art. She went on to use this line of argument to support the use of humanistic research in nursing as a way of linking scientific rigor with the tradition of the art of nursing. She did not, however, suggest that the presence of art in nursing makes nursing an art form.

Peplau (1988) suggests that nursing is an enabling, empowering, transforming art which has the aim of 'moving' people in the same way that they may be moved by music or literature. She suggests that the medium of nursing art is 'the self of the nurse', the process is in nurse–patient interactions, and the outcome is change which is 'primarily interior to the patient' and highly private. This view of nursing art in some ways reflects closely other art forms. For example in painting the medium is paint on canvas, the interaction is between the artist, the paint and the canvas, and the outcome is a painting which elicits individual and private emotions from each observer. An area where nursing does not equate with other art forms in Peplau's explanation however, is that there is a medium other than the artist in art. For painting it is the paint, in music it is the musical instruments, in poetry it is language. Peplau does not identify any medium other than the artist in nursing as art.

In a similar way Diers (1991) suggests that the tool of nursing art is not the body as in dancing, or the voice as in opera singing, but the intellect. However, in enlarging on this idea, her discussion suggests that intellect is not enough because she argues that it is knowledge, for example of electrolyte balance, or dopamine theory, or indeed assessment of circulation to the fingers of a fractured limb, which enables nurses to perform their art. One could equally argue that it is intellect combined with knowledge, this time of colour and perspective, that enables a painter to create a painting. But the painter has tools such as brushes, paints and a canvas. It is the tools of nursing art, beyond intellect and knowledge, which remain unarticulated, thus leaving unanswered the question of whether nursing is an art form.

Despite her discussion of nursing as it equates to art, Peplau (1988), like Watson (1981), asserts that nursing is a science and follows a similar line of argument supporting this view by demonstrating the similarities between science and art in nursing. Thus once again nursing is not being described as fundamentally an art form.

Holmes (1991) enters the debate by confirming that the theory of art and aesthetics is not well developed in nursing. He is explicit in using the philosophical and theoretical underpinnings of art to inform his arguments. He suggests that the primacy of scientific knowledge, and the debate about whether aesthetic knowledge is indeed 'real' knowledge, has led to a focus on research within the paradigms of science, and research based in the philosophy of art being missed along the way.

A major difficulty I encountered in my review of the literature related to nursing and art was the way in which writers seemed to use the terms 'the art of nursing,' and 'nursing as art,' synonymously. This is exemplified by Appleton (1993) who, in seeking to explicate participants' experience of 'nursing when it is art', asked the question 'what is the experience of the art of nursing for you?' This is a problem in art theory, which differentiates between art meaning the product of human skill, and art which holds aesthetic beauty (Stecker, 1993). Where artistry in nursing is discussed, it is usually viewed as the process of caring but which uses science as its tools and thus leads to scientifically measurable outcomes.

Thus I arrived at the stage in my thinking where the seed sown months before was ready to germinate. It was through reflection however that the ground needed to facilitate the germination was made ready. In caring, Mayeroff (1971) suggests that the carer must be able to cope with the caring, must be 'up to' it. Similarly, he suggests, that which is cared for must have the capacity for growth, as a dormant seed has that capacity whereas dead wood does not. Of course, in caring for an idea, it may be that it only becomes apparent that it is dead wood once the process of caring for it has begun.

In caring for the idea, that nursing is an art form, I needed to know that it was an idea capable of growth, and that I could help grow it. The former I felt confident of. I had discussed the idea with various people, including, post-graduate students of nursing, teachers of nursing, educationalists, clinical nurses and also artists and art historians who were not nurses. I received a positive response from all. Nevetheless I was always aware that the idea may turn out to be ungrowable.

The belief that I was 'up to' developing the idea was more difficult. My concept of my intellectual ability, born in childhood, was that I could cleverly play the right game to appear able, and therefore achieve academic qualifications, but that I would one day be found out as a fraud because I was neither analytical nor an original thinker. This belief was not supported by experience in my adult life, such as success in professional and academic examinations. Nevertheless, the childhood 'failures' led me to perceive my adult achievements as somehow fraudulent.

Glover (1988) suggests that our beliefs are so much a part of our identity that they cannot be changed at will. However, he argues that it is through changes of belief that 'self-creation' takes place. I needed to create a new self whom I perceived as capable of growing an idea. Burns (1982, p. 201) asserts that 'it is generally accepted that to modify a person's self-concept to any large extent requires a major act of therapy or some quite traumatic event'. If I was to nurture my idea and help it grow to maturity I had to experience a change of self-concept related to my beliefs about my intellectual ability. It was an unexpected event, which in retrospect could be classified as traumatic, which precipitated the change, and which forms the following critique of personal growth using a reflection cycle (Figure 6.1) to give structure to the process.

◆ **Figure 6.1**   **A Reflection Cycle.**

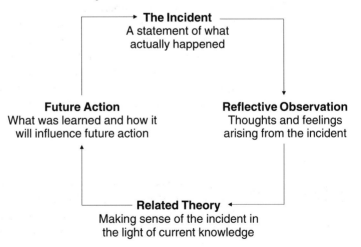

The Incident
A statement of what
actually happened

Reflective Observation
Thoughts and feelings
arising from the incident

Future Action
What was learned and how it
will influence future action

Related Theory
Making sense of the incident in
the light of current knowledge

The incident

I presented a summary of some work I was undertaking and was told by a person present, whose judgement I respect, that I had analysed and synthesized the subject matter well.

Reflective observation

As I presented my work and heard presentations from others in the group, I was aware that I clearly understood my subject, and the processes I had used in my work. I also knew that I compared favourably with the others in the group, some of whom had not yet grasped the nature of the intellectual exercise we were undertaking. When I was told I had shown evidence of analysis and synthesis, by someone I respected, I felt numbed. I knew that synthesis is evidence of independent thinking and I was being told I had done it. The very idea seemed unbelievable, yet I had to believe it or deny the accuracy of the opinion of someone I respected, thus change my belief about her. For a while I felt speechless and those with whom I spent time over the next few hours were aware of my mood, yet I felt unable to share my feelings. As I pondered on this event I became intensely angry. I could no longer know myself as the person who would one day be found out as a fraud. I would have to know myself as intellectually able. Yet, even as I refused to share my feelings with others I knew I could never be the same. I felt so angry at the loss of the self with whom I was familiar. A new self had emerged whom I must come to know. The old self was lost forever and I mourned her.

As I reflected on the numbness, the anger, the knowledge that the old self was gone and that life would never be the same again, I remembered a previous occasion when I had felt similar, though more intense feelings. It was the day that someone very close had died. This added to the trauma, the guilt I felt at linking my present experience with that event. On this occasion however the pain subsided quickly as I began to share the experience and I knew that it was within my power to create a new self out of the loss.

Related theory

In order to make sense of this experience I stepped outside of myself and tried to view it objectively. First I explored why I felt an intellectual fraud. Discussion with colleagues and students revealed that this is not an uncommon feeling. In

129

English culture self-depreciation is a norm and it is not uncommon for children to be taught through constant criticism, that they are of little value. In relation to the development of self, Glover (1988) suggests that self-deception can be a way of maintaining present beliefs about self, rather than taking the harder road of adopting new beliefs. This is perhaps why it takes a cathartic event to stimulate change.

Next I examined the intense feelings I had associated with the loss of my familiar self. Grief theory suggests that with any loss, be it loss of a friend or relative through death, or loss of property through burglary, or loss of life-style through retirement, people go through similar stages of feeling. These stages include denial, shock and disbelief, anger and rage, and finally resolution and acceptance (Kubler-Ross, 1976; Parkes, 1972). Thus I understood that as my experience was one of loss, though perhaps an unusual loss, my strong feelings were to be expected. The plans I made for future action, the final stage of the reflective process, were the way in which I came to resolution and acceptance.

Plans for future action

As an act of respect for the person who stimulated this change, those who helped me during the sort time of trauma, and not least myself, I made an active decision to act always as if I am an intellectually able person. I planned to do this in several ways. First, I decided never again to put myself down in response to a compliment about my work. Secondly, I decided to state my views in any academic debate, referring to my knowledge base as appropriate, rather than keeping quiet for fear of showing myself to be a fraud. Thirdly, I began to think about, and talk about plans for academic study and writing in both the short and long term. Finally I chose to believe that I was up to caring for my idea.

Thus I embarked on a new opportunity for reflection in self-development as I created new incidents by trying out the plans I had made. As I reflect on the occasions when I experimented with this new self, I am aware of feeling both strange, and pleased. Sometimes I fail and slip into the old habits, but as time goes by the new self becomes familiar and the old self fades away. Thus the trauma is being brought to resolution and a change of self-concept is being wrought which will facilitate caring for the idea of nursing as an art form.

Many nurses will be familiar with using a reflection cycle. Before moving on to the next stage in caring for the idea we would like to offer a unique approach to the process of reflection, one which is thousands of years old, and which incorporates an interesting combination of art and science (Kidd, 1992), and when applied to reflection in nursing presents something more than art and science. It is the Socratic Dialogue.

♦

THE SOCRATIC DIALOGUE

Plato (c. 427–347 BC) was both a philosopher and a playwrite in ancient Greece. His philosophy and literary creativity are intertwined and he often expressed his philosophical beliefs and arguments in dramatic literary form. The particular form he used is known as the Socratic Dialogue. Plato took the view that, to present and analyse arguments for personal behaviours, by merely laying out the logical formation of the argument, without taking into account the language or 'literary clothing', would be like looking at a philosophical argument out of focus. Equally, to read his plays without regard to their philosophical direction would not present the whole and would, therefore, be distorted.

Plato used the Socratic Dialogue to present a dramatic play. The combination of art and science in the Socratic Dialogues makes the Dialogue an interesting and unique way to examine reflection in nursing and the nature of nursing knowledge. The scientific paradigm is concerned with objectivity and, indeed, one of Plato's aims in the Socratic Dialogues appears to be the pursuit of objective truth. The chief character in all of Plato's Socratic Dialogues is Socrates, and in all the Dialogues, Socrates seems to suggest that there is certain infallible knowledge or moral truth. On the other hand, the literary aspect of the Socratic Dialogues is an art form, and as such, is characterized by the subjective response of the individual audience or reader. In the Socratic Dialogues, Plato (intentionally or otherwise), created this subjective response in both the characters within the dialogue and amongst philosophy scholars since 347 BC.

The Socratic Dialogues are short plays written by Plato

which contain several characters, one of whom was always Socrates, Plato's mentor and friend who was executed in Athens in 399 BC. The words spoken by the character Socrates in the dialogues, however, are Plato's interpretation of Socrates. It is also worth noting that Socratic Dialogues are neither biographical reporting, nor pure fiction and drama. Rather, according to Kidd (1992), they are 'philosophical faction', which, according to the *Oxford English Dictionary* (1978) is a fictional development from a base of real people, events or situations. The most important thing to understand about the Socratic Dialogues is that they were written, created and directed by Plato in a purposeful way.

The central feature of all Socratic Dialogues is Socrates asking certain questions of various contemporaries. All Socrates does in the dialogues is to ask questions. If we look at Johns' model for structured reflection (1993) we see that, he too, asks questions; indeed, whatever model for reflection is used, it always involves asking questions. Whether Johns' approach to reflective practice can be called a modern day list of Socratic questions is debatable. In any event the character of Socrates merely asks questions of the other characters to enable them to examine their own moral and social beliefs, standards and practices. In this way, the Socratic Dialogue could be seen as an ancient Greek model for reflective practice!

Through the questions asked by Socrates, other players are forced to examine (and reflect on) their beliefs and actions. In the Socratic Dialogue, the person who is being questioned has the option to answer personally, and is capable of saying 'yes' or 'no'. The directive force of the play is the questions (and as many teachers of nursing know, it is not always easy to ask the right questions). Plato's character of Socrates always professes ignorance as he asks his questions.

An illustration of a Socratic Dialogue

One of Plato's earliest and shortest Socratic Dialogues is called *Laches*. It could be described simplistically as a drama of characters where the beliefs of two generals, Laches and Nicias, are examined and tested. It can also be described as a dynamic dramatic philosophical dialogue which has been written, produced and directed by Plato, where he uses his chief character (Socrates) to explore a problem all of us (including Plato) must face: courage.

The theme of courage in this particular Socratic Dialogue

develops over time. The drama unfolds around two fathers, Lysimachus and Melesias, who are anxious about their sons' education. There is a new lecturer in town, Stesilaus, who is teaching weapon drill to young men. The two fathers are discussing whether they should spend their money for their sons to attends Stesilaus' lessons. They decide to consult their two friends, Laches and Nicias, both of whom are famous and successful generals who, they believe, can help them decide.

Nicias, who is quite an enthusiastic follower of the new intellectual enlightenment happening in Greece, is all in favour of sending the two sons to be taught by Stesilaus. His argument is that one skill leads to another, and studying under Stesilaus will lead eventually to the lads becoming generals themselves. Laches, on the other hand, is a practical soldier and is sceptical. He has seen Stesilaus in actual battle, and watched him make a pig's ear of it. Laches also argues that mere technical skill is not enough in a heated battle. What has happened is an impasse, which is a characteristic of Plato's Socratic Dialogues, so the anxious fathers turn to the character of Socrates who is always hovering, like a fly on the wall, in such circumstances, and ask him to give the casting vote.

As you would expect, Socrates does not give an answer. Instead he starts asking his questions. A modern day rendition of the Socratic questions (and answers) in this drama might look like this:

SOCRATES	Would you actually settle this, or any other important issue, simply through a majority decision? Or would you rely on the advice of one expert who knows and who is right?
	No reply from either father.
SOCRATES	Do we know what we are talking about in this situation?
LYSIMACHUS	(Impatiently) Weapon training, of course.
SOCRATES	But isn't that just a means to an end? If we are discussing which eye ointment to apply or not, isn't it the condition of the eyes that we are really concerned about?
MELESIAS	What then is this about?
SOCRATES	Are we not talking about weapon training in relation to the end product of your sons' education? and isn't that end product the care of their minds and moral goodness? *(Here Plato has written in a rather leading question to move the characters on from physical to mental/intellectual/ moral education.)*

133

Silence from the two fathers.

SOCRATES   Isn't moral goodness too large a question. Why don't we confine it to say manliness and courage? Is that all right? *(Although Socrates makes no statement, the nature of the questions are crucial. If the discussion or dialogue is to proceed, he needs agreement from the other characters to proceed. The characters can answer 'yes' or 'no' to the above.)*

As a result of the above, the two generals, as supposed experts, agree to be questioned by Socrates on the subject of courage. Laches agrees to go first and is full of confidence.

SOCRATES   If you know what a thing is, can you say what it is?
LACHES   Absolutely!
SOCRATES   So can you say what courage is?
LACHES   No problem. A man who stands fast in the ranks and fights off the enemy is brave.

Plato has a field day with this kind of question. Plato's philosophical belief is that in attempting to define something, we can go astray in two different ways: firstly, we can set about our definition in the wrong way and get the form of the answer wrong: secondly, the content of our answer can be wrong (Kidd, 1992). Laches definition of courage is wrong because it is not a definition, it is merely an example (x is courageous behaviour rather than courage is x). Socrates convinces Laches of the narrowness of his answer by producing contrary examples (in question form):

SOCRATES   Is it not true that Spartacus broke ranks at the battle of Plataea and won the battle? Is it true that courage has a wide field and can cover illness, poverty, affairs of state, pain, fear or even desires and pleasures? *(This is a contrary example question.)*
LACHES   Oh, well, yes, I suppose so. Let me put it another way. I think courage is a sort of mental endurance; its having guts; bottle. *(Here he's got the form right, e.g. 'courage is x'. But has he got the content right?)*
SOCRATES   Would you accept all 'guts' as courage?
LACHES   Well, no, maybe that's too broad.
SOCRATES   Isn't courage a fine thing?
LACHES   Intelligent endurance is a fine thing but foolish endurance isn't; it's hurtful and possibly vicious. Therefore, foolish

endurance cannot be courage and therefore, intelligent endurance is courage.

(Socrates lets this slightly flawed reasoning go; he's happy to consider it a working hypothesis but he's got some question about what 'intelligence' means.)

SOCRATES   Intelligent is what? Is a city stockbroker who is insider dealing and knows that by buying shares and holding out he will make a lot of money. Is such behaviour courage?

(Also a contrary example question.)

LACHES   No.

SOCRATES   What about a doctor who knows that he will kill his patient if he gives in to his pressure for a drug, and so intelligently sticks out against it?

(Another contrary example question.)

LACHES   No, again, that's not courage.

SOCRATES   What about this then. Two armies are facing each other in battle. The general of one army knows that reinforcements are coming, that hc outnumbers the enemy, and that he is in a stronger position. He clearly sticks it out intelligently. But the other general, knowing the odds are stacked against him, would he not be foolish to stick it out?

LACHES   The second general is brave to stick it out but not the first.

SOCRATES   Are you not saying that the more foolish, or stupid 'guts' constitutes courage? Are you saying that intelligent 'guts' – knowing the odds are with you – isn't courage after all?

What follows is a discussion of how uncomfortable Laches is when his beliefs have come under scrutiny. But more important, the reader notices how the questions Plato has written for his character, Socrates, is focusing attention on the rather puzzling mental aspect of 'guts' in courage – just guts, just sticking it out, is not apparently, enough. Laches retires a bit hurt and frustrated.

Enter Nicias, the second general, who has been listening with interest and although he thinks he's got a clever answer for Socrates, he too falls foul of Socrates' questions as the rest of the drama unfolds.

What has been presented here was a small part of one of Plato's Socratic Dialogues in a 20th century format. It is important to remember that this is a fictitious reflection on a real dilemma, that is, the nature of courage. All the characters and questions are in the mind of the thinker, in essence, in a Socratic Dialogue, the individual questions her or himself. Thus, the purpose of the questions Plato has written into the drama for his character Socrates to ask, is to probe, direct and guide – to challenge thoughts and beliefs; in other words, to reflect. What the *Laches* dialogue does, is to show through the Socratic questions, that the answers offered by the generals are incompatible with previously held beliefs. In the process of answering the questions, Laches and Nicias are reflecting on beliefs about courage and they are learning to clarify and understand what courage really means. A personal knowledge is being developed which, coincidentally, is one of the outcomes of reflecting on practice as described by Schon (1987) and others some 2000 years later. So, in effect, the Socratic Dialogue format was possibly the earliest recorded form of reflection during and after action.

Having described the Socratic dialogue approach to reflection we will return to caring for the idea that nursing is an art form. One of the features of caring for an idea, according to Mayeroff (1971) is to look at it from differing points of view, and Silcock (1991) suggests that non-conformity, that is, thinking in unusual ways, is a mark of creative thinking. I began my exploration of nursing as an art form in the unconventional setting of an art gallery, the National Gallery in London. My intention was first, to examine my feelings as an audience of art, and secondly, to see if art in the form of painting gave me any clues to nursing as art.

This reflection is described in the form of a play, with three scenes, in which the actors are myself, and myself as Socrates. It is a true, but fictionalized, account of an incident. The order of events has been altered in order to create a coherent whole. For example, I did not refer to literature while at the gallery, but afterwards. However, this fictionalization is in keeping with the notion of Socratic Dialogue as a tool to aid reflection.

Scene 1: The Italian Renaissance Gallery

I have wandered round the Gallery looking at each picture briefly. I have now stopped in front of 'The Annunciation with Saint Emidius' by Carlo Crivelli.

MYSELF

Yet another annunciation painting. Nothing different, they are all red, blue and gold, with Mary kneeling, gazing at a human-looking angel.

SOCRATES	Are you looking at it from the right distance? Is there nothing else in it?

I move closer.

MYSELF	It's just a lot of complicated, rather fussy detail.
SOCRATES	Is that what the painting is about, fussy detail?
MYSELF	Well, there's the usual dove, and halo....
SOCRATES	Is there nothing else?
MYSELF	Ah, I see an apple, and a peacock, and some bread. They just seem to be put in randomly, but I hardly noticed them at first. They blend into the picture so they don't seem out of place.
SOCRATES	Blended together? If I put different fruits and fluid in my food processor, they are blended, but the result is a sticky mess. Is this artistic?
MYSELF	Hmm.... I see that the picture is more than just an angel telling Mary she is to have a baby. I need some help here. I'm not sure what it all means?

I turn to my art book (Hall, 1974) and look up the items depicted in the painting. I discover that each is a symbol which has a recognized meaning in the world of art. The dove is the symbol of the Holy Ghost, the halo signifies sanctity, the apple symbolized the fall of man and the mission of Christ. Bread is Christ's sacrifice, and the peacock, his resurrection and immortality.

MYSELF	I see it now. Through the use of symbols this picture tells how the child which Mary will bear, through the intervention of the Holy Ghost, is sinless and will sacrifice Himself for the sins of fallen man, and will rise from the dead for the salvation of humankind.
SOCRATES	Isn't this too general and religious? Why don't we examine it in terms of nursing? Is that all right? *(Seeking approval to continue.)*
MYSELF	Yes, after all that's why I came. I think that nurses nowadays tend to dismiss ritual and routine as having little value in nursing (Walsh and Ford, 1989). Perhaps there is another way of looking at it. For a patient who is largely self-caring, it may seem strange if a nurse approaches apparently simply for a chat, but if she approaches apparently to take a temperature, the patient may recognize that nursing is happening, and be open to conversation. Thus the ritual of taking a temperature may sometimes have a symbolic meaning which then enables other aspects of nursing to occur.

Scene 2: The French Impressionist Gallery	I am standing a foot or so away from Monet's 'Waterlilies'.
MYSELF	All I see is a blurr, meaningless brushstrokes.
SOCRATES	Are you looking at it from the right distance?
	I step backwards.
MYSELF	Ah! This is stunning. A hazey lake, bathed in yellow light, and there floating on the surface, waterlilies, flowering red and white.
SOCRATES	A hazey lake, yellow light and waterlilies are stunning? Are they not just normal elements within nature? *(A contrary example question.)*
MYSELF	What's stunning is not the elements themselves, it's what has been created from them. At first I was confused. I wondered what I was looking at. It made no sense. But stepping back to view the whole, I am amazed at the beauty and integrity of the picture, and it imparts to me a sense of calmness. This is the real painting. The brushstrokes on their own are nothing.
SOCRATES	Is integrity and beauty a good thing then? May we talk about beauty and integrity in nursing? *(Seeking approval to continue.)*
MYSELF	Yes, it leads me to question whether nursing can be viewed as isolated incidents, such as the care of the little boy with the fractured arm described earlier (p. 124 and 125), or does one only see the art if one views the whole. Perhaps the care of the little boy, by both nurses, was only a part of the art created by the whole team of nurses, in the whole ward. Perhaps the less creative nurse was just one brushstroke, and represented the 'shadow' nurse (see Chapter 4). The creative nurse was another brushstroke, and represented the 'archetype' who would perhaps have been invisible had the shadow nurse not been present.
Scene 3: Sitting on a bench in a random gallery	
SOCRATES	If you know about beauty can you say what it is?
MYSELF	I am struck by the whole atmosphere. The light, the peace,

the quiet bustle as people wander from room to room. I feel a sense of beauty that is greater than the paintings on the walls.

SOCRATES   Is it not true that people bustling from room to room can be distracting and annoying, however quiet they try to be? *(A contrary example question.)*

MYSELF   That is not always true. Sometimes it is reassuring. Here the people are part of what makes the gallery what it is.

SOCRATES   And what about you then, sitting on the bench. Where do you fit in?

MYSELF   Ah, I see. I am one of the people too. So I am part of what makes the gallery what it is.

SOCRATES   May we talk about nursing now? There is a lot of bustle and noise as nurses do things to patients. Isn't that quite unlike an art gallery? *(Another contrary example question.)*

MYSELF   I am reminded of my experience in hospital following major surgery. I remember being in considerable pain, but looking round the ward and feeling a deep sense of contentment because I knew I was safe. Somehow the pain ceased to matter as I absorbed the safety of the ward. This notion of the whole of nursing as art is summed up by Lumby (1991), as she admonishes nurses who deny their art, saying, 'I see this art every time I walk into an environment where a nurse is busy "creating" the day for another person. They are busy using light, space, sound, words, movement and touch to deliver the message of care.'

SOCRATES   Is this not art at its finest in nursing?

The curtain falls and I emerge from my visit to the gallery, and my dialogue with Socrates.

Through reflection I discovered that it is possible that nursing is an art form, but I had a new question. I wanted to know more about the philosophy and theory of art. I wanted then to explore nursing practice in relation to art theory to try to give more substance to the idea that nursing is an art form. These explorations form the basis of Chapter 2 and constitute the next stage in caring for my idea.

In caring for my idea, using reflective processes, new thoughts and questions emerged and become more formed. I am growing increasingly confident that the subject can be examined in a more rigorous way. In evaluating the use of reflection in caring for the idea I return to my initial thoughts. I was drawn to the idea of nursing as art through an awareness of a missing element in my understanding of nursing. This led to the idea it might be found in an exploration of nursing as art. A change in my self-concept, through reflection, enabled me to begin this exploration confidently.

At the moment the proposition that nursing is an art form is an idea that I hold. Nursing was the phenomenon which I began to ponder on, and a nuance of my experience of nursing which I could not articulate, was the source of the idea that nursing could be an art form. Using Munhall's (1993) idea of the cyclical continuum described earlier, the next stage in caring for the idea would be to propose a theory and test it using recognized and appropriate methods.

If it can be demonstrated, that nursing is an art form, using reliable evidence which the nursing profession believes, then it will become part of the knowledge base of the discipline of nursing (Adams, 1993). This would constitute a qualitative change in thinking, away from nursing as science to nursing as art. It would therefore have implications for how nurses view their practice, and how nursing is taught at all levels. One would need to question, for example, whether a Bachelor or Master of Arts in nursing be more appropriate than a Bachelor or Master of Science, and whether nursing as an academic discipline be more appropriately situated in humanities faculties than science faculties within universities. The idea is, however, a long way from becoming knowledge.

This chapter has discussed reflection in relation to current literature, and has proposed some different ways of approaching and using the process. However reflection is a dynamic process, often depicted as cyclical. It would therefore be inappropriate to suggest that the ideas proposed here are complete. Indeed they will never be complete. Each of you, in reading this chapter, are engaging in an event upon which you may choose to reflect, or not. If you do, then you will move on the thinking, in directions of your own, creating spin-offs. The spin-offs of the thinking in this chapter are Chapters 2, and 7. Another is the book as a whole. We challenge you to create you own spin-offs and thus move forward your own thinking and practice.

CHAPTER 7   *The picture is nearly complete, as far as any picture can be complete. I feel you have tied things together really well.*

CHAPTER 6   *But this cannot be the end of the story. There are always spin-offs, new directions to travel, because reflection tells nurses that their capacity to learn is endless.*

CHAPTER 7   *Yes, I agree, but nurses must constantly revisit and review their ideas and practices. Reflection offers the means to do this.*

CHAPTER 6   *Quite, they must retain all that is good, but move on from those ideas which at present are no more than academic rhetoric, and are outside the experience of nurses and patients.*

CHAPTER 7   *The old faces of the cube are always there, and make up a part of the whole. It is now time to turn the cube again and reveal a new face....*

A NEW VIEW OF NURSING: TURNING THE CUBE

Pat Rose and Diane Marks-Maran

The previous chapters have offered new ways of thinking about and explaining nursing. Because our capacity to learn and grow is endless, there will always be new directions to travel and new spin-offs to explore.

This chapter will begin by examining existing world views of nursing, where they come from and the extent to which they do or do not influence nursing practice or patient care. This will be presented by examining the perspective of the patient, the perspective of the practising nurse and the perspective of the academic nurse. We will question whether these three world views are similar or different and, more important, whether a nursing world view can be a *world view* if not all the players (scholar, practitioner, patient) share that view?

We will move on from this to propose a new world view, a hitherto hidden face to the cube, which might connect the patient's perspective, the practising nurse's perspective and the academic perspective of a world view, or paradigm, of nursing. This new face to nursing will not, indeed could not, replace or negate all other paradigms of nursing, but it attempts to reconcile the perspectives of all those involved – patient, practitioner, academic.

◆

THE PERSPECTIVE OF THE PATIENT

Whilst considerable effort has gone into the development of models, theories and paradigms in nursing, there is little evidence that the perspective of the patients of nursing has been sought. In reviewing the literature related to caring, McKenna (1993a) identified a number of studies which sought the view of patients and nurses using the same data collection tools for the two groups. The findings are interesting in that the studies reviewed reveal that nurses and patients have differing views of what caring behaviour is. Nurses consistently gave highest ranking to expressive behaviours of nursing such as 'attentive listening', 'comforting', 'honesty' and 'patience'. The ability to perform physical care competently did not appear on the nurses' list of caring behaviour. Conversely, patients gave highest ranking to the instrumental behaviours such as knowing how to give injections and manage equipment, and giving good physical care. McKenna (1993a) went on to suggest explanations to account for these differences.

One explanation is that nurses are socialized, through the education process, to believe that caring equates to expressive behaviours rather than clinical skills. Another explanation she suggests, is that nursing attracts the type of individual who values expressive behaviours above practical skills, and cites studies which indicate that nurses gain great pleasure from these activities. A third explanation is that nurses under-value practical skills because they take them for granted. In other words, nurses see practical care as nursing and the expressive skills as going beyond this. Thus, when nurses are asked about caring behaviours, as opposed to nursing, they will talk about these expressive behaviours. Conversely, patients under-value expressive skills because they are invisible and assumed, whereas the physical nursing actions are what they perceive as receiving care.

Milburn et al (1995) report on a study conducted to examine patients' responses to the question: 'What would you like from a nurse?' Whilst this study did not ask patients to rate behaviours in the way that McKenna's study did, it is interesting to note that, in this study too, physical care was important to patients. In all the studies described here, another factor, as well as physical care, was viewed as important. That was that nurses should be knowledgeable and not only know what they are doing but also be able to give information and provide explanations.

Despite the evidence that physical care is important to

patients, some still argue that, to define nursing in this way, demonstrates a narrow perspective. Castledine (1994) states that 'hard-core traditionalists believe that all nursing is about helping patients with their basic functions and keeping strictly to current rules and principles of hygiene'. Our fear, however, is that if nurses do not do these things as a matter of priority, then patients may be left in wet beds, remain unwashed for days on end, may not be protected from the risks of hospital acquired infection, and so on. This is not to say that the expressive behaviours are unimportant, simply to suggest that the importance of physical care, so valued by patients, must not be under-estimated and must not remain absent in a world view of nursing.

Castledine (1994) makes a valiant attempt to define nursing based on nurturing. He returns to the derivation of the word *nurse*, meaning to nourish, as a mother nourishes a new-born baby, and from there links the word to concepts such as cherishing, fostering, hoping, promoting growth and understanding. He then uses a thesaurus to make further links and comes up with a definition as follows: 'Nursing is nurturing people with their health-related experiences, problems and concerns.' He goes on to list a series of behaviours equating to nurturing. Whilst including assisting, he omits 'doing' from the list. Yet we have already seen, from the research, that patients rate physical activities of nursing highly, and nurses possibly take them so for granted that they do not figure in a nurse's perception of caring or within the articulated paradigms.

In the wake of the UKCC (1994) proposal of three levels of practice, McGee (1993) illustrated the role of the nurse at each level of practice using wound care as an example. She identified what nurses would be expected to know and understand with regard to, for example, types of dressings, healing processes, principles of asepsis and so on. She even suggested that at one level nurses would be able to advise patients, and at another level to advise nurses, about wound care and how to change dressings. But at no point did she suggest that nurses would be able to actually carry out the procedure of dressing a wound, using all the knowledge and understanding they were supposed to have.

♦

One of the major issues in the current nursing world view, or paradigm, is the suggestion that there is a gap between theory and practice. Lindsay (1990) describes this as 'the "great divide" between those who think about doing and those who actually do'. This theory–practice gap is traditionally discussed in relation to nurse education with the 'theory' students are taught in school differing widely from the reality that happens in practice. Lindsay (1990) calls this the negative view, and suggests that its supporters appear to believe that current practice is best practice and that it therefore does not need to be changed or developed, and is what students should be taught. One could argue, however, that this is not so much a negative view as a realistic one. Greenwood (1984) highlighted the failure of nursing research in saying that 'the aim of nursing research is to improve nursing practice, and yet it consistently and spectacularly fails to do so.' Ten years later English (1994) confirms this. He examined 22 years of nursing research and found that it has generally failed to influence practice. He goes on to suggest many possible reasons for this such as, nurses do not know about research, they do not understand or believe the findings, they do not know how to apply them, they are not allowed to use them, they are not relevant to their practice, or they are contradictory.

Whilst suggesting that to be a research-based profession nursing practice must be underpinned by empirically derived theory, and that this is necessary to eliminate practice-based routine and ritual, English (1994) makes some rather contradictory statements himself. First, for example, he suggests that some routine or ritual practices may be contradicted by empirical research, but also that there is an over-abundance of research findings, and that some of them conflict with each other. He then omits to acknowledge that there may be value in ritual (as discussed in Chapters 2 and 6). Secondly, he argues that practice needs to be research-based, but acknowledges that less than a third of published research is deemed useful for guiding practice. This, he suggests, may be because researchers have not asked, and do not know, what clinical nurses want from research. He goes on to make a profound statement of caution to nurse academics: 'If nursing practice can be shown to deliver acceptable standards of care without utilising research findings, then the value of academic nursing itself may be scrutinised.' The suggestion is not that current practice is necessarily best practice but that research offers nothing better. Radcliffe (1995) echoes this view, asking why nursing should be scientific anyway. He suggests concentrating on the non-quantifiable experiences of patients such as emotion and fear rather than empirical research.

Another view of the theory–practice gap is that it is essential to practice development. Lindsay (1990) suggests that this is the positive view because it is theory which is constantly setting new goals for practice. He argues that the thinking practitioner will welcome practice scrutiny and will willingly change in the light of good theory, developed from a position of awareness of current practice. The problem, as we have already seen, is that comparatively little research seems to fulfil this requirement.

Both these schools of thought suggest that there must be, or needs to be, a theory–practice gap. There is, however, one school of thought that suggests that the gap can be closed through the process of reflection: a subject which was fully addressed in Chapter 6. It is enough here then to remind ourselves that reflection is a structured process of examining practice with the purpose of learning from experience, and identifying new ways of practising in the future. The theory–practice gap is closed by using knowledge from theory to gain an understanding of the practice incident concerned and incorporating ideas, both from theory and the experience of practice, into future practice. This is a very individual way of applying theory and research to practice and is, perhaps, more appropriate than an institutional approach, as it recognizes and engages professional autonomy and personal accountability for practice, and the uniqueness of patients.

With regard to human uniqueness, it is important to remember here that the concept of individualized care, to which reflective practice lends itself particularly well, is closely associated with the concept of holism. Holism in relation to nursing is the idea that the individual who is being cared for is a whole, integrated being, who cannot be reduced to parts which can be treated separately. Some nursing world views suggest that holism means looking at all parts of a person, e.g. their biological needs, psychological needs, their social needs and so on. This might mean that the whole person is considered, but not in a holistic way. Any system which separates a person into parts, or systems, is by nature reductionist. Likewise, patient-focused care, which incorporates the concepts of managed care, care maps,

♦ Table 7.1	**The terminology of patient-focused care.**

Term	Description
Managed care	The determining of a multi-disciplinary path of care for each patient, based on medical diagnosis (RCN, 1992, 1994)
Care map	The path of care associated with each medical diagnosis, which provides a framework for every discipline to follow (map being an acronym for Multidisciplinary Action Plan) and which managers agree to resource. It states outcomes and predicts achievement period (Laxade and Hale, 1995)
Multiskilling	Members of all health care professions are trained in certain skills, in order to reduce job demarcation and time wasting (Buchan, 1995). For example, a radiographer may cannulate a vein to give a dye, or a nurse may cannulate and take blood for routine tests (Alderman, 1993)

multi-skilling and evidence-based practice (Table 7.1) might sound holistic and patient-centred, but is in reality a reductionist approach in which care protocols are taken off the shelf and possibly adapted to take into account individual idiosyncrasies.

Thus, any world view of nursing, or model for practice, or care delivery system which derives from such a world view, which addresses, for example, activities of living, or self-care needs, as separate parts of the whole person is not a model which espouses holism. Holism considers all of the person as one, and every person as unique. Thus it is not possible to approach holistic care delivery from a purely rationalistic perspective.

There is increasing emphasis today on the need for nursing, and indeed all health care, to be based on good clinical evidence (NHS Executive 1993, 1994). The evidence used may include: clinical guidelines, patient and public choice, epidemiological information, outcomes (success or failure) of certain interventions, performance measures, organizational audit outcomes and financial audit outcomes. It will be supported by nurse education based on scientific evidence and research, and clinical guidelines, a series of which have been commissioned by the NHS Executive (von Degenberg, 1996).

It is interesting to note that, whilst public and patient choice might be admissible as evidence on which to base practice, the experience of nurses is not listed. Yet a review of some accounts of the use of reflection in practice development reveals that nurses are incorporating theory into practice as part of a creative approach to nursing rather than through adherence to rigid protocols recommended in the context of evidence-based practice and managed care. Parker et al (1995) give an account of a student's learning through reflection, in which the student incorporates theory of communication in her practice, and Ganner (1996) describes the development of her practice in intensive care nursing through incorporating theory associated with critical care nursing. In both cases practice development is through the individual, and will probably only ever be measurable in the experience of future patients of these nurses. Nevertheless, if one views nursing as a practice discipline in which the care of patients is our prime concern, then this is probably the most valuable evidence of quality in nursing. Additionally, the place of intuition is noticeably absent from the list of that which constitutes evidence.

In Chapter 5 intuition was examined and it was clearly argued that, although intuitive decisions cannot be measured quantifiably, there is evidence to suggest that intuitive decisions are often right decisions and that intuitive knowledge is a legitimate form of knowledge upon which to base practice decisions.

One area where there is strong evidence of the positive effect of nursing is in the evaluation of nurse-led care. A report on the initiative at King's Healthcare Trust (Griffiths and Evans, 1995) found that patients cared for by nurses did better than a similar group cared for by doctors, that there was a saving in acute bed usage and a four-fold reduction in routine medical reviews. Garbett (1996) reports on the growth of nurse-led care in both the hospital and community settings. In this era of the promotion of evidence-based practice, nurses need to grasp the opportunity and press for the evidence of the therapeutic effects of nursing to be acted upon, by advocating nurses as the leaders in care delivery.

◆

THE PERSPECTIVE OF THE ACADEMIC NURSE

For the past three decades, a great deal of energy from nursing academics has been put into attempts to clarify the plethora of pseudoscientific terminology that has crept into scholarly publications: terms such as theory, concept, paradigm, domain, framework, model and their derivatives and extensions. McKay (1969) addressed the terms theory, model and system and within that exercise discussed taxonomies, paradigms and phenomena. Torres and Yura (1975) aimed to clarify the meaning and functions of concepts and theories. Keck (1989) reviewed some 15 terms and their associated terminology. For example, in attempting to clarify the term concept she also discussed enumerative concepts, associative concepts, relational concepts, statistical concepts, and summative concepts. It is no wonder then that by the 1990s a full volume of discursive definitions, in the form of a dictionary of nursing theory and research, was needed (Powers and Knapp, 1990).

Cody (1994) has argued that there is a need for a language particular to the discipline concerned, and rejects the call for a language that is easily understood by lay people and members of other disciplines, using the argument that all disciplines have their own language. She adds that 'if there were no room for a new language in science, then there would be no room for new ideas'. She goes on to argue that the reason nurses themselves often oppose nursing theory is that they do not know it. She suggests that the teaching of nursing is often based in other disciplines, sociology, psychology and so on, and that many teachers of nursing do this because they hold degrees and doctorates in those disciplines as opposed to nursing. She adds that nursing theory is the lifeblood of nursing, and that nurses must learn to speak its language.

Perhaps the reason for the lack of clarity has its roots in the nature of nursing as a practice discipline into which the language of science and academia has been transplanted. Of course, there is nothing wrong with enlarging a vocabulary as the understanding of a discipline expands. However, the simultaneous use of jargon in several different ways simply adds confusion. A simple example is in the use of the word *theory*. Hunink (1995, p. 19–20) suggests several meanings for the word as follows:

1. knowledge from books, instructions and guidelines for the practical situation;

2. as the opposite of 'practice' ('in theory' meaning 'not in practice');
3. as a possible explanation, guess, assumption or hypothesis;
4. a way of looking at something, a vision;
5. scientific meaning, e.g.:
    –   a theory as a 'law,' a universal rule (e.g. the law of gravitation);
    –   as an explanation of a number of related facts;
    –   empirically tested knowledge, or knowledge to be tested.

Most nurses will be familiar with the way in which student nurses report that what they do when in college is theory, using the first or second of the definitions above. Constant use of the term in this way means that the fifth, or scientific meanings are subsumed, and attempts to read scientific papers are confused by misunderstanding. This confusion arising from the use of a word differently in different contexts is just one example of confusion in terminology.

More problematic perhaps is the use of terminology in different ways within the same context particularly if that context is academic writing. The example of the word theory given above also illustrates this. Within academic writing any one of the scientific meanings could be intended, or indeed one of the other four meanings. With some of the jargon prevalent in the language of nursing science, this confusion of meaning is so complex that it is difficult to know where to begin. An example is in the terms: person, environment, health and nursing. We all recognize what they are when grouped together, but even as we write we do not know what to call them. Fawcett (1978, 1984b) at different times, calls them units, phenomena and concepts. Manley (1991) suggests that they should more properly be termed constructs. Kershaw (1992) calls them core components. Cameron-Traub (1991) calls them elements. It seems to us that they are merely words which convey different meanings to different people. Grouped together, however, they have come to represent what is known as the metaparadigm of nursing: and that is another word – metaparadigm.

A metaparadigm is defined as representing the world view of a discipline, that is, the most global perspective that subsumes all views and approaches to the concepts of concern (Powers and Knapp, 1990). Put simply, one could say that a metaparadigm is that which all those involved would agree provides a view of the discipline concerned. Thus, in nursing, if all concerned agree that person, environment, health and nursing (which we will henceforth call the four concepts as best representing what they are and for want of a better term, though we seriously thought of calling them *the four words*), represent the discipline of nursing, then it can justly be termed the nursing metaparadigm. Whether this is indeed the case, however, needs to be more fully examined. If a metaparadigm is the world view, or view of all concerned regarding a discipline, then it seems legitimate, as we have attempted to do in this chapter, to examine nursing from the perspective of all those concerned: patients, practising nurses, nurse academics.

We saw earlier that which makes up the patient's world view. We also explored a number of components of the world view of the practising nurse. Now we are engaging in an examination of the world view of the nurse academics; a world view of language and jargon which is often inaccessible, not only to the lay person, but to many practising nurses as well. We begin our exploration with the origins of the four concepts and how they came to be accepted as the metaparadigm of nursing.

The story begins in the 1970s in the USA. Yura and Torres (1975) describe a survey they conducted on behalf of the National League for Nursing Council of Baccalaureate and Higher Degree Programs which had, in 1972, included in its curriculum appraisal criteria, the criterion that curricula should be based on a conceptual framework. The purpose of the survey was 'to identify concepts commonly held by nursing faculty and the terms in which they are expressed' (p. 20). The method used was to identify 50 nursing education programmes which articulated a conceptual framework and obtain self-evaluation reports, which frequently consisted of diagrammatic representation followed by narrative. Each was analysed to identify the components, themes, topics and threads that made up each curriculum. These data were then grouped according to similarities and commonalities. Four major concepts were identified which, it is claimed, were common to all the programmes reviewed. They were: man, society, health and nursing.

By the time Fawcett (1984b) first proposed that the four concepts (man and society by now substituted by person and environment) constituted a metaparadigm of nursing, she claimed that there was already a consensus that this was the case. She supported this by citing 11 sources which made reference to the concepts as central to the domain of nursing. Indeed, she goes on to state that no literature revealed any contradiction. From this time there has been increasing acceptance of the claim that the nursing metaparadigm consists of the person, the environment, health and nursing as its key concepts. Sometimes the claim is accepted without question. Kershaw (1992, p. 104), for example, boldly states: 'All nursing models recognise the core components of man, environment, health and nursing.' Others are as confident. Indeed, in less than a decade, the assertion was being made that there was general agreement amongst nurses regarding the position of the four concepts in nursing theory building (Flaskeraud and Halloran, 1980). Cameron-Traub (1991, p. 36), however, is more circumspect, suggesting that they 'have been identified as components of a possible metaparadigm for nursing.'

It is easy to see that, if an idea is presented as generally accepted, more and more of those concerned will begin to accept it too. Brodie (1984) describes Fawcett's (1984b) proposal that the four concepts constitute the metaparadigm of nursing, as an evolutionary stage, in the spirit of Darwinian evolution and survival of the fittest. At that time, she was referring to the four concepts as the fittest of a whole range of concepts used by nurse theorists to delineate nursing. However, time has perhaps proved her right in that, whilst the proposal has been criticized and other world views have been proposed, none has survived in the way that this one has.

The first criticism of Fawcett's (1984b) metaparadigm is associated with the way it came into being and became labelled as a metaparadigm. By examining nursing models, or conceptual frameworks, to identify the presence of the four concepts, Fawcett (1984b) looked at only one aspect of the discipline of nursing. She did not, for example, review nursing practice in the search for commonality of concepts. Nor is there any evidence that she looked at nursing theory for practice such as theory of pressure area care, or assessment of conscious level. Neither did she seek to find the patient's world view of nursing. Surely, if a metaparadigm is to be proposed, it must be recognizable in all aspects of the discipline it claims to be a world view of. As Brodie (1984) put it, 'Dr. Fawcett addressed only selected concepts and themes of particular theories that would fit into the preconceived formulation,' and it is evident, from our summary of the history of the emergence of the four concepts, that there was indeed a preconceived formulation. This criticism, however, is not enough of itself to suggest that the four concepts do not constitute nursing's metaparadigm, only the evidence would be needed from a much wider variety of theory, practice and patient sources before this can be affirmed.

Another criticism which Brodie (1984) made was that Fawcett (1984b) did not explain the interactions between the four concepts. Fawcett (1993b) has, subsequently, addressed this by drawing on the work of Donaldson and Crowley (1978) and Gortner (1980) to describe four propositions which link the concepts. However, this part of the metaparadigm has not become 'generally accepted' and is often not mentioned by those referring to the metaparadigm (Manley, 1991; Hunink, 1995).

The criticism of any attempt to explicate a metaparadigm within a discipline must include a discussion of the paradigmic level of the discipline's knowledge. A paradigm has been defined as a 'disciplinary matrix' in which there is a shared understanding of the concepts which constitute the metaparadigm (Fawcett, 1984b). In the context of nursing, and using the four concepts, a paradigm is an agreement amongst a group of members of the discipline regarding the definitions and relationships of the concepts, and the theory and practice emerging from and supporting that agreed view. There have been several attempts to identify the paradigms which inform the discipline of nursing.

Fitzpatrick and Whall (1989) suggest that nursing theory may be underpinned by either an organismic world view or a mechanistic world view or by a mixture of both. The organismic view they characterize as focusing on the whole, where the person and the environment are considered an open system, where growth and development can be predicted but the course it takes cannot. The mechanistic view, on the other hand, suggests that the person is separate from the environment and that predictable change will occur in response to stimuli from the environment.

Parse (1987) identifies the paradigms differently. She suggests a simultaneity paradigm in which people are viewed as more than the sum of their parts, they are in mutual rhythmical interchange with the environment, and human experience is a process of becoming within a set of values. As the other view point she suggests a totality paradigm where people are viewed as bio-psycho-social beings who interact with the environment by manipulating it in the striving towards optimal health.

Through careful reading and a struggle through the jargon, it is possible to see that both Fitzpatrick and Whall (1989) and Parse (1987) see nursing theory being generated and proposed from different philosophical bases. They then analyse a series of conceptual models to demonstrate the paradigms they have identified, but they do not analyse any other type of nursing theory, nor do they analyse practice.

The whole point of identifying paradigms is not to decide which is 'right' and which is 'wrong' but to make explicit the philosophy and assumptions which make up the way of looking at the world. Paradigms are simply different ways of looking at the same thing, different faces of the same cube and, at any given time, one of these ways of thinking will be face up and the others face down or facing other ways. We see this in the different paradigms which make up the domain of science: empiricism, historicism and critical science, to name but a few. They are in competition in as much as one may represent majority thinking and, therefore, be viewed as science, at any given time. In the same way paradigms of nursing represent different ways of looking at nursing and compete for dominance. In her proposed metaparadigm and in other works, Fawcett (1984, 1993a, 1993b) seeks to reconcile these opposing paradigms, an unnecessary and inappropriate task.

One of the ways in which nursing practice has been incorporated into Fawcett's (1984b) metaparadigm has been in response to another criticism, that of the inclusion of the *concept* of nursing within the *metaparadigm* of nursing. This is tautology. In simple terms, tautology is the use of a term or concept within a definition or explanation of that term or concept. Thus, to define an apple pie as a 'pie made with apples' is tautologous as it defines neither pie nor apples. In the same way, to say that nursing is a concept of the metaparadigm of nursing is a tautology. Fawcett herself (1993b) has acknowledged the charge but she counters it by saying that because, in the context of the metaparadigm, nursing stands for nursing activities or nursing action, it is not a tautology. However rather than resolving the problem she has created a new tautology. By including this tautology within the metaparadigm of nursing, it cannot be a metaparadigm. One cannot say that a part of what one generally accepts as nursing is nursing.

Other attempts beside Fawcett's have been made to define

a metaparadigm for nursing. Kim (1987), for example, identified a typology of four domains in an attempt to classify the essential concepts of nursing. She later termed this a metaparadigm (Kim, 1989). Her domains were as follows:

1. The patient domain, with the emphasis on knowledge of human phenomena such as ageing and women's health, within a nursing perspective.
2. The patient–nurse domain, defined as phenomena arising out of encounters between the nurse and the patient. Examples given are the individuals involved in the encounters, the social context, the nature of the encounter and the health outcomes.
3. The practice domain, addressing phenomena associated with the cognitive, behavioural and social aspects of nursing actions, such as decision-making, competence and development of expertise.
4. The environmental domain, addressing not only factors such as time and space but also issues such as information transmission systems and collaboration with other health professionals.

Another alternative is proposed by Ramos (1987). She suggests that the search for a metaparadigm of nursing is the wrong approach; an unrealistic expectation given that nursing is an ever-changing discipline in which practice responds to environmental and social change. If this is the case, then the central concerns of nursing will be determined, not by the direction of the emergent or agreed metaparadigm, but must reflect current practice. She introduces to nursing the ideas of Toulmin (1972), who suggests that the intellectual endeavours of a discipline should be directed towards problems which arise from the practice arena. In the light of this view, Ramos (1987) suggests that, rather than striving for a metaparadigm, meaningful activities in nursing research would be: to evaluate how well nursing knowledge solves practice problems; to refine nursing language and understanding of concepts in order to communicate more meaningfully; to explore ways in which the behavioural repertoire of nursing can be transmitted to a novice to promote development of expertise; and to address all these areas in the light of tacit as well as overt knowledge.

It is interesting to note that, despite the attempt to demonstrate that nursing actions and activities are included in Fawcett's (1984b) metaparadigm, this is the viewpoint which addresses practice least well; yet it is the one that has been most widely accepted. The alternatives described above have both fallen by the wayside. One of the reasons for this may be that the term 'metaparadigm' is generally better understood in the scientific context by academics and that science is more highly valued than other forms of knowledge in academia. Perhaps it should more properly be called the metaparadigm of nursing science. Indeed, there is a school of thought that argues that the existence of a discipline, as a body of knowledge, is separate from the activities of the practitioners (Donaldson and Crowley, 1978) and which would, presumably, argue that there must, therefore, always be a theory–practice gap.

Conway (1985) suggests that these two fields, theory and practice, are associated with conceptual frameworks of nursing, and caring, respectively. She goes on, however, to argue that, whilst the discussions related to whether nursing has a metaparadigm or an agreed paradigm will have little influence on the development of nursing's body of knowledge, there needs to be consensus regarding the metaparadigm. This, she suggests, is necessary in order to establish the central concerns of nursing and, thus, the direction of nursing research, rather than rely on an individual researcher's personal views as to what are the important questions for nursing.

Several issues emerge from the preceding discussion. Firstly, there is less consensus amongst nurse academics regarding the four concepts constituting a world view of nursing than the literature at first suggests. Secondly, that existing explanations of a world view of nursing may actually demonstrate that there is no one agreed world view and, thirdly, the world views as described by nurse academics contain concepts and language which make them inaccessible to the other two groups of people who have a stake in the discipline of nursing: practising nurses and patients.

◆

A NEW FACE ON THE CUBE

The metaphor of the cube has been the thread throughout this book. It was selected by us merely as a way of portraying that there are different ways of viewing nursing;

no matter how you turn the cube, one face will always be totally visible, others partially visible and others will be hidden.

Nursing is a practice discipline. Without the reality of nurses doing nursing, there is no nursing discipline. Additionally, without the reality of nurses in relationship with patients, there is no nursing discipline. It is clear too, that the knowledge (scholarship) of nursing cannot be separated from its practice. Practice is scholarship in action; scholarship is the thought and knowledge behind the practice. The two are not opposites in conflict but rather they are valuable together or, as Wolinsky (1994) would say, they are opposites which are made of the same substance and are, therefore, not in conflict with each other.

Nursing scholarship is less about what a nurse knows and more about how a nurse thinks, acts and is. The new face of nursing – a new nursing world view – suggests that the kinds of thinking which constitute nursing scholarship are precisely the kinds of thinking which constitute practice as it takes place. In addition, the being and doing of nursing which constitute intuitive, caring nursing practice are precisely the kinds of being and doing which constitute nursing scholarship. The concepts which make up the face of the cube are, therefore, as follows:

- ◆ critical thinking and practice;
- ◆ reflective thinking and practice;
- ◆ creative thinking and practice;
- ◆ moral thinking and practice;
- ◆ intuitive thinking and practice;
- ◆ doing, knowledgeably and wisely;
- ◆ caring;
- ◆ being in relationship with patients.

Any analyses of nursing scholarship and/or nursing practice will be based on these concepts. There is art and science within each of these concepts and yet each is more than the sum of its art and science.

The notion of combining nursing scholarship with nursing practice is a deliberate one. Verena Tschudin (Chapter 4) described Wolinsky's (1994) explanation of chaos theory concluding that, rather than concentrating on opposites as being different, opposites are seen to be made of essentially the same substance. When opposites are viewed in this way, any conflict about them dissolves and problems between them disappear. This, according to Wolinsky, is true integration. Nursing has viewed theory and practice as opposites in conflict. Indeed, the notion of a theory–practice gap which widely appears in the literature, begins from a premise that theory and practice are opposites in conflict. Instead, chaos theory allows us to concentrate on theory (scholarship) and practice in terms of the energy which flows between them.

The new world view of nursing – new face of the cube – which we offer here is based on just this: there is energy created between nursing scholarship and nursing practice, between the art of nursing and the science of nursing, between theory and practice. By exploring – and embedding ourselves in – the flow of energy between the two, we gain our own energy. But Verena Tschudin also suggested in Chapter 4 that we can often be afraid of the chaos which is caused by being asked to change from adherence to one end of a spectrum considering the possibility of that which is on the opposite pole of the spectrum. If we are primarily engaged in nursing practice, we cling to the safety of that which is practice, resisting or rejecting nursing theory as an irrelevance. If we are primarily engaged in nursing scholarship, we condemn those whose practice does not reflect theory and scholarship. This view of scholarship and practice, art and science, as being opposite are a part of previous paradigms of nursing.

What is being proposed here is a new world view of nursing which invites us to experience the energy between the two and be energized by it. Rather than concerning ourselves with conflict between the two, we focus our attention on the energy between them. And this energy sharpens our critical thinking, makes us responsive to our reflections, fosters creativity, builds moral purpose, enhances our capacity to be in a relationship with patients, creates caring and enables us to tap into our intuitive selves. All of the concepts within our new world view of nursing are touched by the energy we receive when we cease to view science and art as opposites in conflict. We can give a name to this energy. Its name is nursing. The new world view of nursing moves away from previous paradigms, based on disconnected concepts in the abstract, towards a connectedness world view based on energy processes. This is essential nursing 'reconstructed' as described by Jean Watson (Chapter 3).

As we move away from the notion of theory and practice as opposites as being strictly dualistic, we reconstruct nursing reality into a new world view. Pat Rose (Chapter 2) suggests that nursing is not nursing theory or science or technology. Instead, nursing is that which the nurse creates using this knowledge and tools of theory, science and technology. In essence, nursing is then creative energy which bridges art and science. The new paradigm being proposed suggests that nursing scholarship and nursing practice are a part of the same substance. Each nurse as artist will be unique in the way she creates artistic nursing through engaging in the activities within the paradigm, and each member of the audience of the art (patients) will find meaning in the nurse's artistry, and healing energy from it which will be unique to that individual. Table 7.2 illustrates the concepts and connections of the new paradigm.

To enhance clarity, a paradigm, or world view, of nursing needs to be examined through exploring cases which occur both within the paradigm and outside it. The illustration presented in Chapter 6 about the young boy who had returned from the operating theatre following an operation to reduce his fractured arm provides examples of a case occurring both within and without the new paradigm. Re-read the account on pages 124–125. On the one hand there was the nurse who demonstrated nearly all the attributes of the new world-view, critical thinking in practice, creativity, morality, intuition, knowledgeable and wise nursing actions, caring and being in relationship with her young patient. The outcome was that she gained what information she needed (the fingers of his hand were pink and warm) but also gained his trust, calmed his fears, demonstrated compassionate relationship through creatively combining observation of his fingers with human touch.

The case occurring outside the paradigm demonstrated nursing within a different face of the cube, a rationalistic face, where the object of gaining the empirical data (colour and warmth of fingers) was of paramount importance, with little evidence of creativity. It demonstrated dubious moral thinking and behaviour, caring more for the data which needed to be collected than for the child, and was devoid of any obvious relationship between the nurse and her patient to facilitate completion of the nursing task. Both nurses involved obtained the information they sought but they did so within two opposite world views of nursing. The first worked in a way which demonstrated the connection between task and relationship, thinking and doing, creating, measuring and science. The connection was not between

◆ Table 7.2 Concepts and connections in nursing practice and scholarship: a new paradigm.

Concept	Opposites	Connections
Critical thinking and practice	Care planning and care giving are based on assessment, evidence analysis, and a rational justification for decisions.	Evidence and action can come from science, technology, research, reflection-in-action, intuition and creativity.
Reflective thinking and practice	Reflecting-before-action involves seeking evidence to justify decisions; reflecting-in-action leads to responsiveness to feedback as an action is taking place; reflection-on-action is learning from recent experience to better inform future practice. Flexibility is built into nursing practice to take into account changing realities.	Reflection is nursing scholarship to inform practice; the process uses evidence and generates evidence; leads to 'ah ha' experiences which are often intuitive and largely creative; leads to doing knowledgeably and wisely.
Creative thinking and practice	Unique change in a patient's physical, emotional, social and/or spiritual state resulting from nursing actions; the explicit understanding and recognition of the unpredictability of being human and, therefore, the unpredictability of nursing.	The nurse is more than one who does; the nurse creates the environment for the caring–healing relationships and conditions for all other concepts to be manifest; thinking, being and doing in extraordinary ways.
Moral thinking and practice	Patient autonomy, choice and best interests are facilitated; a moral dimension influences decision-making; practice is influenced by ethical purpose, part of the 'being' of nursing.	Morality is about our notions of right and wrong, good and bad; it therefore underpins the whole search for nursing scholarship and the seeking to act in the patient's best interests; all other concepts are, in part, moral concepts.

Intuitive thinking and practice	Knowing without being able to give reason; incorporating tacit knowledge and data gained from experience; generating questions from 'hunches' to create new scholarships, making a good practice decision which you cannot explain.	Intuition is an additional type of evidence to be critically analysed, reflected upon, trusted. The nurse taps into intuition processes through her relationships with patients and through touching the soul of the patient; intuition leads to creative decisions and actions.
Doing knowledgeably and wisely	Undertaking the caring manual tasks of nursing with an understanding of how, why and when.	Instilling confidence in patients through doing tasks with creative use of manual skills; the bringing together of all other concepts when undertaking a nursing task.
Caring	Connecting with your patient; the soul of the nurse touching the soul of the patient; the artistry of feelings, compassion and aesthetics.	Caring is morality in action; it is also the manifestation of intuition and creativity in nursing; caring provides the environment for science, technology and critical thinking to take place.
Being in relationship with patient	Establishment of a therapeutic relationship which contributes to body-mind-spirit healing; part of the 'being' of nursing.	Any therapeutic relationship which contributes to healing involves something greater than the sum of all the concepts together. All of the concepts together create, recreate and enhance the therapeutic nurse–patient relationship.

opposites in conflict but rather opposites made of the same substance, joined together by an energy we call nursing.

♦

SUMMARY

When we move away from viewing art and science in a conflicting, dualistic way, we invite a new world view or paradigm for nursing, a new face of the cube. We propose here that chaos theory as interpreted by Wolinsky (1994) offers a new way of seeing art and science in nursing as being made of the same substance. Rather than continue to resist the chaos caused by viewing the opposites in conflict (art vs. science) in nursing, we can instead concentrate on the energy between the two and the flow of energy between art and science. Whatever new patterns emerge will reveal a 'new nursing' or just nursing.

When we called the first pages of this book *The Beginning* that was not strictly true. This chapter and the book end here, but for you and for nursing, if what was proposed is not wrong (Bach, 1978), it is really only the beginning....

References

Adam E (1987)   Nursing theory: what it is and what it is not. *Nursing Papers* **19**(1): 5–13.

Adams F (1993)   Epistemology. In: McHenry L & Adams F (eds) *Reflections on Philosophy: Introductory Essays*. New York: St. Martin's Press.

Albarran JW (1995)   Should nurses be politically aware? *British Journal of Nursing* **4**(8): 461–465.

Alderman C (1993)   Ceaseless change. *Nursing Standard* **7**(29): 18–20

Allan JD and Hall BA (1988)   Challenging the focus on technology: a critique of the medical model in a changing health care system. *Advances in Nursing Science* **10**(3): 22–34.

Appleton C (1993)   The art of nursing: the experience of patients and nurses. *Journal of Advanced Nursing* **18**: 892–899.

Argyris C and Schon D (1974)   *Theory in Practice: Increasing Personal Effectiveness.* Massachusetts: Addison-Wesley.

Atkins S and Murphy K (1993)   Reflection: a review of the literature. *Journal of Advanced Nursing* **18**: 1188–1192.

Bach R (1978)   *Illusions: Adventures of a Reluctant Messiah*. London: Pan Books.

Barnum BJS (1994)   *Nursing Theory: Analysis, Application, Evaluation.* Philadelphia: Lippincott.

**Bastick T
(1982)**
Intuition: How We Think and Act. New York: John Wiley.

**Begley A-M
(1995)**
Literature, ethics and the communication of insight. *Nursing Ethics* 2(4): 287–295.

**Behi R and
Nolan M (1995)**
The nature of scientific knowledge: fact or theory? *British Journal of Nursing* 4(4): 221–224.

Benner P (1984)
From Novice to Expert: Excellence and Power in Clinical Nursing. Menlo Park, CA: Addison-Wesley.

**Benner P and
Tanner C
(1987)**
Clinical judgement: how expert nurses use intuition. *American Journal of Nursing* 87(1): 23–31.

**Benner P and
Wrubel J (1989)**
The Primacy of Caring: stress and coping in clinical nursing. Menlo Park, CA: Addison-Wesley.

**Bergstrom N,
Braden B,
Laguzza A and
Holman V
(1987)**
The Braden scale for predicting pressure sore risk. *Nursing Research* 36: 205–210.

**Bergum V
(1994)**
Knowledge for ethical care. *Nursing Ethics* 1(2): 71–79.

**Bevis EM
(1989)**
The curriculum consequences: aftermath of revolution. In *Curriculum Revolution: Reconceptualising Nursing Education*, pp. 115–134. New York: National League For Nursing.

Birx E (1993)
Critical thinking and theory based practice. *Holistic Nursing Practice* 7(3): 21–27.

Boleni J (1979)
The Tao of Synchronicity and the Self. San Francisco: Harper and Row.

**Bond S and
Thomas LH
(1991)**
Issues in measuring outcomes of nursing. *Journal of Advanced Nursing* 16: 1492–1502.

**Boud D, Keogh
R and Walker
D (eds) (1985)**
Reflection: Turning Experience into Learning. New-York: Kegan Page.

Boyd CO (1993) The philosophical foundations of qualitative research. In: Munhall P & Boyd CO (eds) *Nursing Research: A Qualitative Perspective*, pp. 66–93. New York: National League for Nursing.

Bradshaw A (1994) Critical Care. *Nursing Times* 90(40): 28–31.

Brink PJ (1993) The art and science of nursing. *Western Journal of Nursing Research* 15(2): 145–147.

Brodie JN (1984) A response to Dr. J. Fawcett's paper: 'The metaparadigm of nursing: present status and future refinements'. *Image: Journal of Nursing Scholarship* 16(3): 87–89.

Brophy GH, Carey ET, Noll J, Rasmussen L, Searcy B and Stark NL (1994) Hildegard E. Peplau: Psychodynamic Nursing. In: Marriner-Tomey A (ed.) *Nursing Theorists and Their Work*, pp. 203–218, 3rd ed. St Louis: Mosby.

Buchan J (1995) Are patient-focused hospitals working. *Nursing Standard* 10 (8): 30.

Bullough V and Bullough B (1979) *The Care of the Sick: The Emergence of Modern Nursing*. London: Croom Helm.

Burman E (ed.) (1990) *Feminists and Psychological Practice*. Sage: London.

Burnard P (1991) Improving through reflection. *Journal of District Nursing* May: 10–12.

Burns RB (1982) *Self-concept Development and Education*. London: Holt, Rinehart and Winston.

Callahan D (1994) Bioethics: Private Choice and Common Good. *Hastings Center Report* 24(3): 28–31.

Cameron-Traub E (1991) An evolving discipline. In: Gray G & Pratt R. (eds) *Towards a Discipline of Nursing*, pp. 31–49. Melbourne: Churchill Livingstone.

Campbell AV (1984) *Moderated Love: A Theology of Professional Care*. London: SPCK.

Carlisle D   MPs to debate need for executive posts (News item).
(1995)   *Nursing Times* **91**(6): 6.

Carper B (1978)   Fundamental patterns of knowing in nursing. *Advances in Nursing Science* **1**(1): 13–23.

Casey A (1988)   A partnership with child and family. *Senior Nurse* **8** (4): 8–9.

Castledine G   A definition of nursing based on nurturing. *British Journal of Nursing* **3**(3): 134–135.
(1994)

Chalmers AF   *What is this Thing Called Science?* 2nd edn. Milton Keynes:
(1982)   Open University.

Chenault J   The scientific facade. *Nursing Outlook* **12**(Oct): 32.
(1964)

Chetwynd T   *A Dictionary of Symbols*. London: Paladin.
(1982)

Chinn PL (1994)   Art and esthetics in nursing. *Advances in Nursing Science* **17**(1): viii.

Chinn KR and   *Theory and Nursing: A Systematic Approach*. 2nd edn, St
Jacobs MK   Louis: Mosby.
(1987)

Chinn PL and   *Art and Aesthetics in Nursing*. New York: National League
Watson J (eds)   for Nursing.
(1994)

Clarke M   Action and reflection: practice and theory in nursing.
(1986)   *Journal of Advanced Nursing* **11**: 3–11.

Clarke M   Memories of breathing: a phenomenological dialogue;
(1992)   asthma as a way of becoming. In: Morse JM (ed.)
                    Qualitative Health Research, pp. 123–140 Sage: London.

Cody WK   The language of nursing science; if not now, when? *Nursing
(1994)   Science Quarterly* **7**(3): 98–99.

Condon EH   Nursing and the Caring Metaphor: Gender and Political
(1992)   Influences on an Ethics of Care. *Nursing Outlook* **40**(1): 14–19.

Conway ME (1985) Toward greater specificity in defining nursing's metaparadigm. *Advances in Nursing Science* 7(4): 73–81.

Conway J (1994) Reflection, the art and science of nursing and the theory practice gap. *British Journal of Nursing* 3(3): 114–118.

Craig S (1980) Theory development and its relevance for nursing. *Journal of Advanced Nursing* 5: 349–355.

Crystal D (ed.) (1990) *The Cambridge Encyclopaedia.* Cambridge: University Press.

Cull-Wilby B and Pepin JI (1987) Towards a coexistence of paradigms in nursing knowledge development. *Journal of Advanced Nursing* 12: 515–521.

Dalai Lama (1995) *The Power of Compassion.* London: Thorsons.

Darbyshire P (1994) Understanding the life of illness: learning through the art of Frida Kahlo. *Advances in Nursing Science* 17(1): 51–59.

Dealey C (1996) The background to the national clinical guidelines for the prevention and management of pressure sores. *British Journal of Nursing* 5(1): 52–53.

Dickoff J and James P (1968) A theory of theories: a position paper. *Nursing Research* 17(3): 197–203.

Diers D (1991) Learning: the art and craft of nursing. *American Journal of Nursing* 91(1): 65–66.

Docking S (1993) Developing reflective practice skills. *Professional Nurse* October. Pull-out supplement.

Doering L (1992) Power and knowledge in nursing: a feminist post-structuralist view. *Advances in Nursing Science* 14(4): 24–33.

DOH (1994) Clinical supervision for the nursing and health visiting professions. *CND Letter* 94(5). London: HMSO.

Donaldson SK and Crowley DM (1978) The discipline of nursing. *Nursing Outlook* 26(2): 113–120.

Douglas D and Robb A (1995)	Clarifying outcomes in clinical practice. *Nursing Standard* 9 (24): 29–30.
Ellis R (1982)	*Advances in Nursing Science* (editorial) 4(4): x–xi.
English I (1993)	Intuition as a function of the expert nurse: a critique of Benner's novice to expert model. *Journal of Advanced Nursing* 18: 387–393.
English I (1994)	Nursing as a research-based profession: 22 years after Briggs. *British Journal of Nursing* 3(8): 402–405.
Eraut M (1985)	Knowledge creation and knowledge use in professional contexts. *Studies in Higher Education* 10(2): 117–133.
Fawcett J (1978)	The 'what' of theory development. In: National League for Nursing (ed.) *Theory Development: What, Why, How?* pp. 17–33. New York: National League for Nursing.
Fawcett J (1984a)	*Analysis and Evaluation of Conceptual Models of Nursing.* Philadelphia: F.A. Davis.
Fawcett J (1984b)	The metaparadigm of nursing: present status and future refinements. *Image: Journal of Nursing Scholarship* 16(3): 84–87.
Fawcett J (1993a)	From a plethora of paradigm to parsimony in world views. *Nursing Science Quarterly* 6(2): 56–58.
Fawcett J (1993b)	*Analysis and Evaluation of Nursing Theories.* Philadelphia: F.A. Davis.
Ferguson M (1980)	*The Aquarian Conspiracy.* London: Paladin.
Field P (1987)	The impact of theory on the clinical decision making process. *Journal of Advanced Nursing* 12: 563–571.
Fitzpatrick JJ and Whall AL (1989)	*Conceptual Models of Nursing: Analysis and Application.* London: Appleton and Lange.
Flaskerud JH and Halloran EJ (1980)	Areas of agreement in nursing theory development. *Advances in Nursing Science* 3: 1–7.

Forrest D (1989)   The experience of caring. *Journal of Advanced Nursing* **14**: 815–823.

Friedson E (1971)   *Profession of Medicine: A Study of the Sociology of Applied Knowledge.* New York: Dodd Mead.

Freire P (1972)   *Pedagogy of the Oppressed.* Harmondsworth: Penguin.

French (1992)   The quality of nurse eductaion in the 1980s. *Journal of Advanced Nursing* **17**: 619–631.

Gaarder J (1995)   *Sophie's World.* London: Phoenix House.

Ganner C (1996)   Using reflection in a critical care unit. *Nursing Standard* **10**(15): 23–26.

Garbett R (1996)   The growth of nurse-led care. *Nursing Times* **92**(1): 29.

Gendron D (1994)   The tapestry of care. *Advances in Nursing Sciences* **17**(1): 25–30.

Gerrity P (1987)   Perception in nursing: the value of intuition. *Holistic Nursing Practice* **1**(3): 63–71.

Glover J (1988)   *I: The Philosophy and Psychology of Personal Identity.* London: Penguin.

Gortner SR (1980)   Nursing science in transition. *Nursing Research* **29**: 180–183.

Greenwood J (1984)   Nursing research: a position paper. *Journal of Advanced Nursing* **9**: 77–82.

Greenwood J (1993)   Reflective practice: a critique of the work of Argyris and Schon. *Journal of Advanced Nursing* **18**: 1183–1187.

Greipp ME (1996)   Client Age, Gender, Behavior: Effects on Quality of Predicted Self and Colleague Reactions. *Nursing Ethics* **3**(2): 126–139.

Griffiths P (1995)   Progress in measuring nursing outcomes. *Journal of Advanced Nursing* **21**: 1092–1100.

Griffiths P and Evans A (1995)   *Evaluating a Nurse-led In-patient Service: An Interim Report.* London: King's Fund and King's Healthcare.

Gullickson C
(1993)
My death nearing its future: a Heideggerian hermeneutical analysis of the lived experience of persons with chronic illness. *Journal of Advanced Nursing* **18**: 1386–1392.

Haase JE (1987)
Components of courage in chronically ill adolescents: a phenomenological study. *Advances in Nursing Science* **9**(2): 64–80.

Habermas J
(1972)
Knowledge and Human Interest. London: Heinemann.

Habermas J
(1974)
Theory and Practice. London: Heinemann.

Hale C (1995)
Case management and managed care. *Nursing Standard* **9** (19): 33–35.

Hall J (1974)
Dictionary of Subjects and Symbols in Art. London: John Murray.

Hammond P
(1994)
Healing is believing. *Nursing Times.* **90**(40): 55.

Hampton DC
(1994)
Expertise: the true essence of nursing art. *Advances in Nursing Science* **17**(1): 15–24.

Hanford L
(1993)
Ethics and disability. *British Journal of Nursing* **2**(19): 979–982.

Hanks P (ed)
(1990)
Collins English Dictionary (2nd edn). London: Harper Collins.

Hardy ME
(1978)
Perspectives on nursing theory. *Advances in Nursing Science* **17**(1): 37–38.

Harries G
(1995)
Use of humour in patient care. *British Journal of Nursing* **4** (17): 984–986.

Harrison-Barbet
A (1990)
Mastering Philosophy. London: Macmillan.

Hill DW and
Summers R
(1994)
Medical Technology: A Nursing Perspective. London: Chapman and Hall.

Holmes C (1991)	Theory: where are we going and what have we missed on the way? In: Gray G & Pratt R (eds.) *Towards a Dicsipline of Nursing*, pp. 435–460. Melbourne: Churchill Livingstone.
Horton I, Bayne R and Bimrose J (1995)	New Directions in Counselling: A Roundtable. *Counselling* 6(1): 34–40.
Hospers J (1990)	*An Introduction to Philosophical Analysis*, 3rd edn. London: Routledge.
Hunink G (1995)	*A Study Guide to Nursing Theories*. Edinburgh: Campion Press.
Husserl E (1970)	*The Crisis of European Sciences and Transcendental Phenomenology*. Evanston, USA: Northwestern University Press. (originally published in German, 1954).
James S (1995)	Gossip, stories and friendship: confidentiality in midwifery practice. *Nursing Ethics* 2(4): 298–302.
Jarvis P (1992)	Reflective practice in nursing. *Nurse Education Today* 12(3): 174–181.
Johns C (1992)	*Assessment of Practice: Ten Key Characteristics, The Challenge of Reflective Practice*. London: ENB.
Johns C (1993)	Professional supervision. *Journal of Nursing Management* 1(1): 9–18.
Johnson JL (1991)	Nursing science: basic, applied or practical? Implications for the art of nursing. *Advances in Nursing Science* 14(1): 7–16.
Johnson JL (1994)	A dialectical examination of nursing art. *Advances in Nursing Science* 17(1): 1–14
Jones S and Brown L (1993)	Alternative views on defining critical thinking through the nursing process. *Holistic Nursing Practice* 7(3): 71–76.
Jung CG (1933)	*Psychological Types*. New York: Harcourt Brace.
Jung CG (1946)	The fight with the shadow. *Collected Works* Vol 10. London: Routledge & Kegan Paul.

Jung CG (1964)   *Man and His Symbols*. London: Picador.

Jung CG (1969)   *The Structure and Dynamics of the Psyche*, 2nd edn. Princeton: Princeton University Press.

Kahneman D and Tversky A (1982)   On the study of statistical intuitions *Cognition* 1(11): 123–141.

Keck JF (1989)   Terminology of theory development. In: Marriner-Tomey A (ed.) *Nursing Theorists and their Work*, 2nd edn, pp. 15–23. St Louis: Mosby.

Kelly B (1991)   The professional values of English undergraduate nurses. *Journal of Advanced Nursing* 16: 867–872.

Kelpin V (1992)   Birthing pain. In: Morse JM (ed.) *Qualitative Health Research*, pp. 93–103. London: Sage.

Kershaw B (1992)   Nursing models. In: Jolley M & Brykczynska G (eds) *Nursing Care: The Challenge to Change*, pp. 103–137. London: Edward Arnold.

Kidd I (1992)   Socratic questions. In: Gower B & Stokes M (eds) *Socratic Questions: The Philosophy of Socrates and its Significance*. London: Routledge.

Kikuchi JF and Simmons H (1992)   *Philosophic Inquiry in Nursing*. London: Sage.

Kim HS (1983)   *The Nature of Theoretical Thinking in Nursing*. Connecticut: Appleton-Century-Crofts.

Kim HS (1987)   Structuring the nursing knowledge system: a typology of four domains. *Scholarly Inquiry for Nursing* 1(2): 99–110.

Kim HS (1989)   Theoretical thinking in nursing: problems and prospects. In: Akinsanya J (ed.) *Recent Advances in Nursing: Theories and Models of Nursing*. Edinburgh: Churchill Livingstone.

Kim HS (1993)   Philosophy, theory and method in nursing science. *Journal of Advanced Nursing* 18(5): 792–800.

Kim MJ, McFarland GK and McLane AM (1993)
Pocket Guide to Nursing Diagnosis, 5th edn. St. Louis: Mosby.

Kinmouth A (1992)
Managing of feverish children at home. *British Medical Journal* 305(6862): 1134–1136.

Kubler-Ross E (1976)
On Death and Dying. London: Macmillan.

Langer SK (1957)
The Problems of Art: Ten Philosophical Lectures. New York: Charles Scribner.

Langford G (1973)
Human Action. New York: Doubleday.

Lather P (1991)
Getting Smart: Feminist research and pedagogy with/in the post-modern. New York: Routledge.

Lawler J (1991)
Behind the Screens. Edinburgh: Churchill Livingstone.

Laxade S and Hale CA (1995)
Managed care 1: an opportunity for nursing. *British Journal of Nursing* 4(5): 290–294.

Lindsay B (1990)
The gap between theory and practice. *Nursing Standard* 5(4): 34–35.

Loye D (1983)
The Sphinx and the Rainbow. London: New Science Library.

Lumby J (1991)
Threads of an emerging discipline: praxis, reflection, rhetoric and research. In: Gray G & Pratt R (eds) *Towards a Discipline of Nursing*, pp. 461–484. Melbourne: Churchill Livingstone.

McGee P (1993)
Defining nursing practice. *British Journal of Nursing* 2(9): 1022–1026.

McKay R (1969)
Theories, models and systems for nursing. *Nursing Research* 18(5): 393–399.

McKenna G (1993a)
Caring is the essence of nursing. *British Journal of Nursing* 2(1): 72–75.

McKenna G (1993b)
Unique theory – is it essential in the development of a science of nursing? *Nurse Education Today* 13(2): 121–127.

Mackay L (1993)	*Conflicts in Care; Medicine and Nursing.* London: Chapman & Hall.
Manley K (1991)	Knowledge for nursing practice. In: Perry A & Jolley M (eds) *Nursing: A Knowledge Base for Practice*, pp. 1–27. London: Edward Arnold.
Marriner A (1975)	*The Nursing Process: A Scientific Approach to Nursing Care.* St Louis: Mosby.
Marriner-Tomey A (ed.) (1994)	*Nursing Theorists and Their Work*, 3rd edn. St Louis: Mosby.
Martin GD (1990)	*Shadows in the Cave.* Harmondsworth: Arkana, Penguin.
Masson V (1987)	Maggie Jones. *Journal of Christian Nursing* March, 22–24.
May KA (1994)	Abstract knowing: the case for magic in method. In: Morse JM (ed.) *Critical Issues in Qualitative Research Methods*, pp. 10–21. London: Sage.
Mayeroff M (1971)	*On Caring.* New York: Harper and Row.
Maynard A (1994)	Knowledge based – not blindly biased. *Nursing Management* 1(4): 9.
Medawar P (1969)	*Induction and Intuition in Scientific Thought.* London: Methuen.
Meleis A (1991)	*Theoretical Nursing: Developments and Progress*, 2nd edn. Philadelphia: Lippincott.
Menzies IEP (1960)	A case-study in the functioning of social systems as a defense agaisnt anxiety. *Human Relations* 13: 95–121.
Merkle Sorrell J (1994)	Remembrance of things past through writing: aesthetic patterns of knowing in nursing. *Advances in Nursing Science* 17(1): 60–70.
Mezirow J (1988)	A critical theory of adult learning. *Adult Education* (US) 32(1): 3–24.

Milburn M,
Baker M-J,
Gardner P,
Hornsby R and
Rogers L (1995)
Nursing care that patients value. *British Journal of Nursing* 4(18): 1094–1098.

Miller A (1985)
The relationship between nursing theory and nursing practice. *Journal of Advanced Nursing* 10: 417–424.

Mitchell WJT
(1992)
Mute posey and blind painting. In: Harrison C & Wood P (eds) *Art in Theory 1900–1990*, pp. 1109–1111. Oxford: Blackwell.

Moore T (1992)
Care of the Soul. New York: Harper Collins.

Munhall P
(1993)
Epistemology in nursing. In: Munhall P & Boyd CO (eds) *Nursing Research: A Qualitative Perspective*, pp. 39–65. New York: National League for Nursing Press.

Myers I and
Myers P (1980)
Gifts Differing. Palo Alto, CA: Consulting Psychologists Press.

National
Health Service
Executive
(1993)
Improving Clinical Effectiveness (EL(93)115). London: HMSO.

National
Health Service
Executive
(1994)
Improving the Effectiveness of the National Health Service (EL(94)75). London: HMSO.

Neuman B
(1982)
The Neuman Systems Model: Application in Nursing Education and Practice. Norwalk: Appleton-Century-Crofts.

Newell R (1992)
Anxiety, accuracy and reflection: the limits of professional development. *Journal of Advanced Nursing* 17: 1326–1333.

Newell R (1994)
Reflection art, science or pseudo-sciences? *Nurse Education Today* 14(2): 79–81.

Newens A
(1995)
Go on, prove it. *Nursing Standard* 9(26): 51.

Newman MA (1986)	*Health as Expending Consciousness*. St Louis: Mosby.
Newman MA, Sime A and Corcoran-Perry S (1991)	The focus of the discipline of nursing, *Advances in Nursing Science* 14(1): 1–6.
Newman MA (1992)	Prevailing paradigms in nursing. *Nursing Outlook* 40(1): 10–13.
Niebuhr HR (1963)	*The Responsible Self*. San Francisco: Harper & Row.
Niebuhr R (1932)	*Moral Man and Immoral Society*. New York: Charles Scribener's Sons.
Nightingale F (1859)	*Notes on Nursing*. London: Harrison and Sons. Reprinted (1992) Philadelphia: JB Lippincott Company. Commemorative Edition.
Noddings N (1984)	*Caring: A Feminine Approach to Ethics and Moral Education*. Berkeley: University of California Press.
Norton D, McLaren R and Exton-Smith AN (1962)	*An Investigation of Geriatric Nursing Problems in Hospital*. Edinburgh: Churchill Livingstone.
Oakley A (1982)	Interviewing women: a contradiction in terms. In: Roberts H (ed.) *Doing Feminist Research*, pp. 30–61. London: Routledge.
Oakley A (1984)	What price professionalism? The importance of being a nurse. *Nursing Times* 80(50): 24–28.
Oberle K (1995)	Measuring nurses' moral reasoning. *Nursing Ethics* 2(4): 303–313.
Oppenheimer H (1995)	Mattering. Paper delivered at Society for the Study of Christian Ethics. *Studies in Christian Ethics* 8(1): 60–76.
Orem DE (1985)	*Nursing: Concepts of Practice*. 3rd edn. New York: McGraw Hill.

Ornstein R (1972) *The Psychology of Consciousness.* New York: Viking Press.

Packard SA and Polifroni EC (1991) The dilemma of nursing science. Current quandaries and lack of direction. *Nursing Science Quarterly* **4**(1): 7–13.

Parker DL, Webb J and D'Souza B (1995) The value of critical incident analysis as an educational tool and its relationship to experiential learning. *Nurse Education Today* **15**(3): 111–116.

Parkes CM (1972) *Bereavement.* Harmondsworth: Penguin.

Parse RR (1981) *Man-living-health: A Theory for Nursing.* New York: John Wiley.

Parse RR (1987) *Nursing Science: Major Paradigms, Theories and Critiques.* Philadelphia: WB Saunders.

Parse RR (1992a) The performing art of nursing. *Nursing Science Quarterly* **5**(4): 147.

Parse RR (1992b) Human becoming: Parse's theory of nursing. *Nursing Science Quarterly* **5**(1): 35–42.

Parse RR (1994) Quality of life: sciencing and living the art of human becoming. *Nursing Science Quarterly* **7**(1): 16–21.

Parse RR (ed.) (1995) *Illuminations: The Human Becoming Theory in Practice and Research.* New York: National league for Nursing Press.

Pearson A (1983) *The Clinical Nursing Unit.* London: Heinemann.

Peplau HE (1952) *Interpersonal Relations in Nursing.* New York: GP Putnam.

Peplau HE (1988) The art and science of nursing: similarities, differences and relations. *Nursing Science Quarterly* **1**(1): 8–15.

Polit DF and Hungler BP (1991) *Nursing Research: Principles and Methods*, 4th edn. Philadelphia: Lippincott.

Polit DF and Hungler BP (1993)
Essentials of Nursing Research: Methods, Appraisal, and Utilization, 3rd edn. Philadelphia: Lippincott.

Polyani M (1958)
Personal Knowledge: Towards a Post-critical Philosophy. London: Routledge.

Polyani M (1966)
The Tacit Dimension. London: Routledge and Kegan Paul.

Powell JH (1989)
The reflective practitioner in nursing. *Journal of Advanced Nursing* 14: 824–832.

Powers BA and Knapp TR (1990)
A Dictionary of Nursing Theory and Research. London: Sage.

Pyles S and Stern P (1983)
Discovery of nursing Gestalt in critical care nursing: the importance of the grey gorilla syndrome. *Image: Journal of Nursing Scholarship* 15(2): 21–28.

Quinn JF (1994)
Caring for the caregiver. In: Watson J (ed.) *Applying the Art and Science of Human Caring*, pp. 63–71. New York: National League for Nursing Press.

Radcliffe M (1995)
Unimpressive stuff. *Nursing Times* 91(30): 189.

Radice B (1971)
Who's Who in the Ancient World. London: Penguin.

Rafferty C (1987)
An apologist's theories for the nursing profession: adaptation and art. *Nursing Forum* 23(4): 124–126.

Ramos MC (1987)
Adopting an evolutionary lens: an optimistic approach to discovering strength in nursing. *Advances in Nursing Science* 10(1): 19–26.

Reason P and Rowen J (1981)
Human Inquiry: A Sourcebook of New Paradigm Research. Colchester: John Wiley.

Reed J and Procter S (1993)
Nurse Education: A Reflective Approach. London: Edward Arnold.

Rew L (1986)
Intuition: concept analysis of a group phenomenon. *Advances in Nursing Science* 8(2): 21–28.

Rew L and Barrow EM (1987)	Intuition: a neglected hallmark of nursing knowledge. *Advances in Nursing Science* 10(1): 49–62.
Rich A and Parker D (1995)	The ethical and moral implications of using reflection and critical incident analysis in nursing and midwifery education. *Journal of Advanced Nursing* 22: 1050–1057.
Roach MS (1992)	*The human act of caring: a blueprint for the health professions.* Ottawa: Canadian Hospitals Association Press.
Rogers ME (1970)	*An Introduction to the Theoretical Basis of Nursing.* New York: FA Davis.
Rogers ME (1989)	Nursing: a science of unitary human beings. In: Riehl-Sisca J (ed.) *Conceptual Models for Nursing Practice*, 3rd edn. Englewood Cliffs: Appleton and Lange.
Roper N, Logan W and Tierney A (1985)	*The Elements of Nursing*, 2nd edn. Edinburgh: Churchill Livingstone.
Rose P and Parker D (1994)	Nursing: an integration of art and science within the experience of the practitioner. *Journal of Advanced Nursing* 20: 1004–1010.
Rose P, Beeby J and Parker D (1995)	Academic rigour in the lived experience of researchers using phenomenological methods. *Journal of Advanced Nursing* 21: 1123–1129.
Roy C (1981)	*Introduction to Nursing: An Adaptation Model*, 1st edn. New Jersey: Prentice-Hall.
Roy C (1984)	*Introduction to Nursing: An Adaptation Model*, 2nd edn. New Jersey: Prentice-Hall.
Royal College of Nursing (1992)	Differing approaches to nursing care. Issues in Nursing and Health Series. *Nursing Standard* 7(8): 38–39.
Royal College of Nursing (1994)	A guide to setting up patient-focused care. Issues in Nursing and Health Series. *Nursing Standard* 9(3): 29.

Royal College of Nursing and Royal College of Midwives (1993) *Strategey for Research in Nursing, Midwifery and Health Visiting: Annexes 1–4.* London: RCN and RCM.

Salvage J (1990) The theory and practice of new nursing. *Nursing Times* 84(4): 42–45.

Santopinto MDA (1989) The relentless drive to be ever thinner: a study using phenomenological method. *Nursing Science Quarterly* 2(1): 29–36.

Sarter B (1988) Philosophical sources of nursing theory. *Nursing Science Quarterly* 1(2): 52–59.

Savage J (1995) *Nursing Intimacy.* London: Scutari Press.

Schon DA (1983) *The Reflective Practitioner.* London: Temple South.

Schon DA (1987) *Educating the Reflective Practitioner.* London: Jossey-Bass.

Schotter J (1974) *Images of Man in Psychological Research.* London: Methuen.

Schraeder B and Fischer D (1986) Using intuitive knowledge to make clinical decisions *Maternal-Child Health* 11: 161–162.

Scott PA (1995) Aristotle, nursing and health care ethics. *Nursing Ethics* 2(4): 279–285.

Seed A (1991) *Becoming a Registered Nurse; the students' perspective.* PhD thesis, CNAA: Leeds Polytechnic.

Shaw MC (1993) The discipline of nursing: historical roots, current perspectives and future directions. *Journal of Advanced Nursing* 18: 1651–1656.

Sheppard A (1987) *Aesthetics: An Introduction to the Philosophy of Art.* Oxford: University Press.

Silcock P (1991) Learning nursing: what factors are responsible for a lack of creativity. *Nursing Practice* 4(3): 24–28.

Silva MC (1977)   Philosophy, science, theory: interrelationships and implications for nursing research. *Image: Journal of Nursing Scholarship* 9(3): 59–63.

Slater V (1992)   Modern physics, synchronicity and intuition. *Holistic Nursing Practice* 6(4): 20–25.

Smith JP (1981)   *Nursing Science in Nursing Practice.* London: Butterworths.

Smith M (1992)   Is all knowing personal knowing? *Nursing Science Quarterly* 5(1): 2–3.

Smith P (1992)   *The Emotional Labour of Nursing.* Basingstoke: Macmillan.

Smith V (1994)   An ordinary experience. In: Ainley R (ed.) *Death of a Mother*, pp. 1–7. London: Harper Collins.

Stecker R (1993)   Aesthetics. In: McHenry L & Adams F (eds) *Reflections on Philosophy: Introductory Essays*, pp. 103–119. New York: St Martin's Press.

Stewart W (1992)   *An A–Z of Counselling Theory and Practice.* London: Chapman & Hall.

Sweeney NM (1994)   A concept analysis of personal knowledge: application to nursing education. *Journal of Advanced Nursing* 20: 917–924.

Tarnas R (1993)   *The Passion of the Western Mind.* New York: Ballantine Books.

Teasdale G and Jennett B (1974)   Assessment of coma and impaired consciousness. *Lancet* 2 (7872): 81–84.

Thompson CB, Ryan SA and Kitzman H (1990)   Expertise: the basis for expert system development. *Advances in Nursing Science* 13(2): 1–10.

Torrence EP (1964)   *Guiding Creative Talent.* New Jersey: Prentice Hall.

Torres G (1990)   The place of concepts and theories within nursing. In: George JB (ed.) *Nursing Theories: The Base for Professional Nursing Practice*, 3rd edn. London: Prentice-Hall.

Torres G and Yura H (1975)	The meaning and functions of concepts and theories within education and nursing. In: National League for Nursing (ed.) *Faculty Curriculum Development, Part 3, Conceptual Framework – Its meaning and Function*, pp. 1–8. New York: National League for Nursing.
Toulmin S (1972)	*Human Understanding.* New Jersey: Princeton University Press.
Toulmin S (1990)	*Cosmopolis: The Agenda of Modernity.* New York: Free Press.
Tronto JC (1993)	*Moral Boundaries: A Political Argument for an Ethic of Care.* New York: Routledge.
Tschudin V (1995)	*Counselling Skills for Nurses*, 4th edn. London: Baillière Tindall.
Turner T (1992)	The indomitable Mr. Pink. *Nursing Times* 88(24): 26–29.
UKCC (1992a)	*Code of Professional Conduct*, 3rd edn. London: United Kingdom Central Council for Nursing, Midwifery and Health Visiting.
UKCC (1992b)	*Scope of Professional Practice.* London: United Kingdom Central Council for Nursing, Midwifery and Health Visiting.
UKCC (1994)	*The Future of Professional Practice – The Council's Standards for Education and Practice Following Registration.* London: United Kingdom Central Council for Nursing, Midwifery and Health Visiting.
Uris R (1993)	*Post-modern Feminist Emancipatory Research: a critical analyses of nurses moral experience in caring in a patriarchal society.* PhD Dissertation, University of Colorado School of Nursing.
von Degenberg K (1996)	Clinical guidelines: improving practice at local level. *Nursing Standard* 10(19): 37–39.
Walsh M and Ford P (1989)	*Nursing Rituals, Research and Rational Actions.* Oxford: Butterworth-Heinemann.
Waterlow J (1985)	A risk assessment card. *Nursing Times* 81(48): 48–55.
Watson J (1981)	Nursing's scientific quest. *Nursing Outlook* 29(7): 413–416.

Watson J (1984)   *Nursing: Human Science and Human Care.* New York: National League for Nursing.

Watson J (1987)   Nursing on the caring edge: metaphorical vignettes. *Advances in Nursing Science* 10(1): 10–18.

Watson J (1988)   New dimensions of human caring theory. *Nursing Science Quarterly* 1(4): 175–181.

Watson J (1995)   Postmodernism and knowledge development in nursing. *Nursing Science Quarterly* 8(2): 60–64.

Watson J and Ray MA (eds) (1988)   *The Ethics of Care and the Ethics of Cure: Synthesis in Chronicity.* New York: National League for Nursing.

Way C and Segatore M (1994)   Development and preliminary testing of the neurological assessment instrument. *Journal of Neuroscience Nursing* 26 (5): 278–287.

Webb C (1992a)   What is nursing? *British Journal of Nursing* 1(11): 567–568.

Webb C (1992b)   The use of first person in academic writing: objectivity, language and gatekeeping. *Journal of Advanced Nursing* 17: 747–752.

Wescott M (1968)   *Antecedents and Consequences of Intuition.* Poughkeepsie, NY: US Department of Health and Welfare.

Wichowski HC (1994)   Professional uncertainty: nurses in the technologically intense area. *Journal of Advanced Nursing* 19: 1162–1167.

Wolinsky, S (1994)   *The Tao of Chaos: Essence and Enneagram.* Connecticut: Bramble Books.

Yura H and Torres G (1975)   Today's conceptual frameworks within Baccalaureate Nursing Programs. In: National League for Nursing (ed.) *Faculty Curriculum Development, Part 3, Conceptual Framework – Its Meaning and Function*, pp. 17–25. New York: National League for Nursing.

Zornow RA (1977)   A curriculum model for the expanded role. *Nursing Outlook* 25(1): 43.

Index